An
INSIDER'S
GUIDE

to
Physician
Engagement

An INSIDER'S GUIDE to Physician Engagement

Andrew C. Agwunobi

ACHE Management Series

Your board, staff, or clients may also benefit from this book's insight. For more information on quantity discounts, contact the Health Administration Press Marketing Manager at (312) 424-9450.

This publication is intended to provide accurate and authoritative information in regard to the subject matter covered. It is sold, or otherwise provided, with the understanding that the publisher is not engaged in rendering professional services. If professional advice or other expert assistance is required, the services of a competent professional should be sought.

The statements and opinions contained in this book are strictly those of the author and do not represent the official positions of the American College of Healthcare Executives or of the Foundation of the American College of Healthcare Executives.

22 21 20 19 18   5 4 3 2 1

Library of Congress Cataloging-in-Publication Data
Names: Agwunobi, Andrew C., author.
Title: An insider's guide to physician engagement / Andrew C. Agwunobi.
Description: Chicago, IL : HAP, [2018] | Series: ACHE management series |
    Includes bibliographical references.
Identifiers: LCCN 2017022347 (print) | LCCN 2017019804 (ebook) | ISBN
    9781567939200 (Ebook) | ISBN 9781567939217 (Xml) | ISBN 9781567939224 (Epub) |
    ISBN 9781567939231 (Mobi) | ISBN 9781567939194 (print : alk. paper)
Subjects: LCSH: Hospital-physician relations. | Hospitals–Administration. |
    Leadership.
Classification: LCC RA971.9 (print) | LCC RA971.9 .A39 2018 (ebook) | DDC
    362.17/2068–dc23
LC record available at https://lccn.loc.gov/2017022347

The paper used in this publication meets the minimum requirements of American National Standard for Information Sciences—Permanence of Paper for Printed Library Materials, ANSI Z39.48-1984. ♾ ™

Found an error or typo? We want to know! Please e-mail it to hapbooks@ache.org, mentioning the book's title and putting "Book Error" in the subject line.

For photocopying and copyright information, please contact Copyright Clearance Center at www.copyright.com or (978) 750-8400.

Acquisitions editor: Janet Davis; Project manager: Joseph R. Pixler; Cover designer: Brad Norr; Layout: PerfecType

Health Administration Press
A division of the Foundation of the American
    College of Healthcare Executives
One North Franklin Street
Suite 1700
Chicago, IL 60606-3529
(312) 424-2800

HALF
BOOKS

Thank you for your order, Melinda Mills!

Half Price Books
1835 Forms Drive
Carrollton, TX 75006
OFS OrderID   19506151

||||| |||| || ||| ||| ||||| |||| | |||

SKU	ISBN/UPC	Title & Author/Artist	Shelf ID	Qty	OrderSKU
S288632367	9781567939194	An Insider's Guide to Physician Engagement.. 06--04--4 Agwunobi, Andrew		1	

Visit our stores to sell your books, music, movies games for cash.

SHIPPED STANDARD TO:

Melinda Mills
8311 Pennsylvania Run Road
LOUISVILLE KENTUCKY 40228-2176
39scjmz4t3mc5lb@marketplace.amazon.com

ORDER# 113-6788381-1205841
AmazonMarketplaceUS

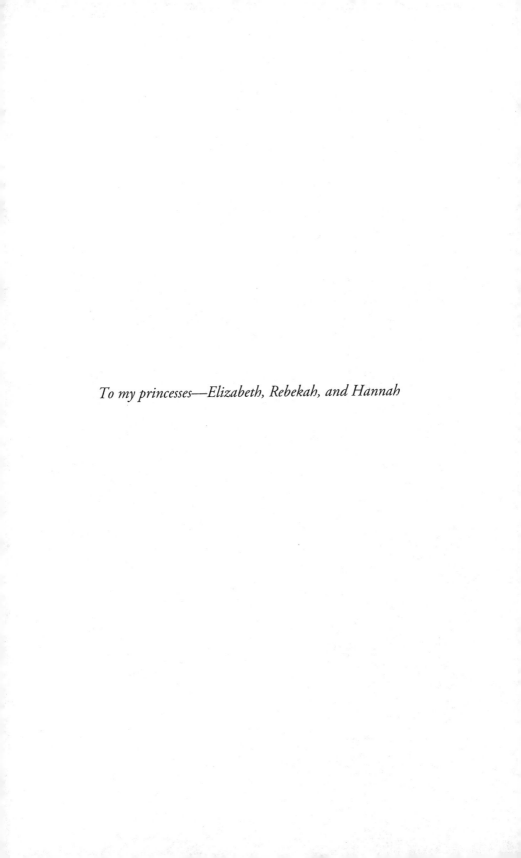

To my princesses—Elizabeth, Rebekah, and Hannah

Contents

Foreword

HEALTHCARE'S SHARE OF the US gross domestic product is expected to rise from 17.8 percent ($3.5 trillion) in 2015 to 19.9 percent ($5.5 trillion) by 2025, according to a 2017 report from the Office of the Actuary at the Centers for Medicare & Medicaid Services. These are staggering numbers. Fortunately, as Dr. Andy Agwunobi shows, it's possible to lower costs while producing better patient outcomes.

The elixir lies in better management and, in particular, de facto physician co-ownership of the challenge. If the considerable capabilities of physicians to help can be harnessed, better care is available at lower costs.

Andy's lessons are those not of an armchair professor but of a highly credentialed medical doctor and health system CEO. His methods are innovative but consistent with what we know about the management of expert talent, and doctors are exceedingly talented individuals with good hearts and capable of much more than is usually asked of them. In his "insider's guide," Andy lays out how activating the cooperation capabilities of physicians can improve the management of a health system. It's not so much a case for getting incentives right—although that matters—but for bringing often-disillusioned physicians into the management process.

But how do healthcare executives get physicians to co-own not just patient outcomes but also operational, financial, and strategic goals? Andy explains how to tap into the altruistic instincts of doctors and their problem-solving capabilities. Part of the solution is for executives to demonstrate an appreciation of the physician's everyday experience by, for example, scrubbing-in with surgeons. The conversion of doctors to coleaders requires organizational respect and recognition for the physician. Physicians are not to be cajoled but rather are to be invited to join the top management team as fellow travelers and treated more as clients than as employees. Putting the doctors first in terms of recognition, respect, and commendation is part of the Andy Agwunobi elixir.

This collaborative, shared-power and shared-responsibility model for management has its origins in Silicon Valley. The allure of Fairchild Semiconductor and Intel in the 1970s was that, for the first time in the electronics industry, the finance gurus from New York City were marginalized and scientist engineers such as Bob Noyce and Gordon Moore were put in charge. This approach was revolutionary for business and is revolutionary in healthcare today as MBA doctor-managers take executive roles in many systems. The Agwunobi approach allows physician leaders to make decisions such as hiring staff, implementing new services, and changing schedules.

Andy maintains that a shift is needed from executives holding all the power to executives sharing the power with physicians, which enables executives to bring necessary transformation to their organizations.

The catnip that stimulates this physician–health executive nexus is data analysis. Data indicate only directional change, but data analysis can help build understanding of problems. Doctors pay attention to evidence; they are used to diagnostic tools in medicine that involve visualization (e.g., CT scans). It is smart to arm them with data that can settle arguments, or at least focus discussion in a meaningful manner. Management approaches that are evidence based, insight driven, and theory informed have a good chance of helping hospitals and health systems simultaneously lower costs and improve patient care.

All this is not easy. But it is possible, and those who adopt the Agwunobi way can help make it happen. We at the Berkeley Research Group are fortunate to have had access to Andy's leadership and experience implementing new approaches. We can attest that it works, and so can the hospitals and health systems that have worked with us.

Today's sharing economy, popularized by Airbnb and apps such as Uber, is about tapping into the physical capital stock that is locked up and underutilized. The fact that the intellectual capital of our doctors has been caged for so long is a pity. The Agwunobi strategy to unlock human capital is, of course, much more than an app, but its benefits are similar. The beneficiaries are patients, doctors, and our overburdened payers—society at large. Let's hope readers will see this ever so clearly and quickly be part of reforming a system desperately in need of a transformation.

Dr. David J. Teece
Institute for Business Innovation, UC Berkeley
Chairman, Berkeley Research Group

Preface

THIS IS THE first book I have published, but the second I have written. My two daughters, 12-year-old Hannah and 14-year-old Rebekah, dismissed my first attempt as "a thousand pages of boring medical stuff." They were right. I spent too much time rehashing hospital industry woes—"admiring the problems," so to speak—and not enough on practical solutions. It was also boring because, in trying to sound intellectual, I lost my true voice: that of a healthcare leader who lives the challenges of my audience every day. Plus, it was way too long.

This book is different. I wrote it because I am passionate about physician engagement and know how to accomplish it. Engaging physicians is the first skill executives must learn and apply to prepare their health systems for the changes ahead.

Over the course of my more than 20 years as a physician, health system CEO, and consultant, I've become convinced that getting physicians to feel *ownership* in the success of their hospitals and clinics is the key to overcoming our challenges in healthcare. I've also realized how hard it is to arrive at physician ownership. There is no precise road map, but the starting point is clear, and that is physician engagement.

Even so, I didn't plan to write this book until a particular physician convinced me. I was telling my wife, Elizabeth, a hospitalist, about a physician engagement initiative I had just implemented in a health system. Elizabeth possesses a natural wisdom that enables her to effortlessly pinpoint flaws in seemingly flawless plans, and to see solutions that have evaded me for days. In other words, she is the brains in our marriage. After listening approvingly (and she doesn't always listen to me approvingly), Elizabeth said, "I wish all healthcare leaders would implement similar initiatives—just imagine the power of doctors and executives working together to improve healthcare."

With those simple words, the clouds parted. The need for a guidebook on physician engagement became clear. With my background and experience—and passion for the subject—I felt compelled to write it.

In this book, I have tried to speak plainly. The best executives I have met are plain talkers who value directness in others. They also value humility born of hard experience and the knowledge that no one has solved all of the tough problems in healthcare. Keeping those executives in mind helped me to stay in my own skin rather than slip into the persona of a professor stroking his beard.

I have also worked hard to keep my recommendations practical. This book is me, an industry insider, telling you, fellow healthcare executives, about what I have implemented, helped to implement, or seen implemented. The examples are all real, although I have modified them to protect confidentiality.

Finally, I kept this book short for healthcare leaders who don't have the time or inclination to read long books. I couldn't get all of my ideas down to a single, "good to great" phrase in the vein of Jim Collins, but at least it's nowhere near a thousand pages.

I hope you will find this book helpful and enjoy reading it as much as I enjoyed writing it. If you do, all credit goes to my wife and daughters.

Andy
Andrew C. Agwunobi, MD, MBA

Acknowledgments

I AM INDEBTED to everyone at Berkeley Research Group (BRG), particularly the Hospital Performance Improvement (HPI) practice. The invaluable consulting experience I gained at BRG helped immensely as I wrote this book. Special thanks to Paul Osborne, the leader of HPI, for his help during the initial writing process and for being a good person and a great friend. I thank Marvin Tenenbaum, Tri MacDonald, and Phil Rowley for their encouragement and support. And I thank David Teece for his wise guidance in the book's early stages, his kindness, and his leadership of BRG—a great role model, indeed.

I also thank Janet Davis and Joseph Pixler of Health Administration Press. Joe, my editor, in particular was a pleasure to work with. He taught me a lot and made the book much better.

Most of all, thanks to my family: my wife, Elizabeth, and daughters, Rebekah and Hannah, for always believing in me and reenergizing me; my mother, for fostering my love of reading and writing, even as she struggled financially; my father, for instilling the importance of knowledge and always setting the bar high; my brother John, without whom my career in the United States and this book would not have occurred; my two sisters, Grace and Anne Marie; and my brother Ignatius. I am so grateful for their love and support.

CHAPTER 1

Recognize Disengagement

PHYSICIAN DISENGAGEMENT HAS been growing inexorably for decades. What's really unfortunate is that physicians have stopped struggling against it; disengagement has become the new normal for physicians just when health system executives need their help the most. The premise of this book is that the solution to most challenges health systems face in today's era of decreasing reimbursement, value-based care changes, and brutal market competition is for executives to engage physicians as coleaders.

COLEADERSHIP

Coleadership goes beyond asking physicians to be partners on specific initiatives, such as reducing length of stay. It means a radical culture change where executives and physicians jointly guide the organization. The premise behind the premise is that health systems, as healing organizations, are best run by both healthcare executives and healthcare providers.

Case in Point: Many years ago, physicians were deeply involved in the leadership of hospitals. In the early 1900s,

$\rightarrow$

the American College of Surgeons (ACS) was responsible for identifying minimal standards for organized medical staffs, accurate medical records, and adequate treatment and diagnostic facilities. ACS later became a founder of the organization that evolved into today's main hospital accrediting body, The Joint Commission.

Fast forward to the present, and such promising beginnings are lost in history. Physicians have relinquished aspirations to be involved in the leadership of health systems, and instead they have withdrawn almost completely to the sphere of treating patients. I would argue that as physicians left the leadership stage, the executive task of optimizing the performance of health systems became impossible.

When I refer to physician coleaders, I don't just mean medical directors or department chairs; I also include rank-and-file doctors. A culture of physician empowerment is impossible unless all physicians feel ownership, because regardless of whether physicians are formal leaders, they lead the care for their patients. Coleadership, therefore, refers to shared leadership between executives and the medical staff.

True, the pendulum of attitudes about physicians as leaders has started to correct. More doctors are being hired as health system CEOs, and in some systems, a dyad model pairs executives with physician leaders to promote a balanced management approach. These are good trends, but they don't go far enough. For example, only 5 percent of health systems have a physician CEO, and in most systems using the dyad model, the culture doesn't change to support true coleadership: The dyads exist, but the executive half of the dyad still leads the physician half (Robeznieks 2014).

I hear less about dyads today. Instead, there is movement toward physician leadership development programs. This evolution is fine, but executives are often confused about what to teach physicians and what to do with them once they are taught. This confusion results from a lack of a clear premise or goal for the leadership development programs and causes many of them to fall short and fizzle out over time.

Coleadership is a difficult concept for many executives, and even some physicians, to embrace. Therefore, it is hard for health systems to achieve. It's difficult for executives to embrace because not only must they share power, they also must share power with a group that is indifferent (at best) or antagonistic (at worst). For physicians, coleadership is difficult because they feel so marginalized and disengaged that the concept of leading anything outside of direct patient care is inconceivable.

For both sides, the challenge is compounded by a lack of trust. In fact, trust between executives and physicians has eroded so completely that what I once described as abutting silos are now distinct workforces separated by a demilitarized zone.

Although hard to accomplish, the concept of coleadership is simple to describe: Executives must share decision making with physicians, while physicians must take responsibility for the success of the whole health system.

Shining examples of physician authority and accountability still exist. One such example is Mayo Clinic. As John H. Herrell, chief administrative officer of Mayo Clinic from 1993 to 2001, observes in *Management Lessons from Mayo Clinic* (Berry and Seltman 2008, 102):

> What differentiates Mayo Clinic is the structure that makes the physician accountable for what happens throughout the institution. If the institution fails, the physicians have only themselves to blame. This fact affects physician behavior at Mayo Clinic in a positive way. They must keep the institution's interests in mind because those interests are aligned with their own.

Creating such a structure and culture isn't easy; Mayo Clinic has the advantage of having been founded by physicians more than 100 years ago and it still isn't perfect. The good news, however, is that just as fallow land can eventually produce bountiful crops, even health systems that have never engaged their physicians have the potential to achieve unimagined levels of success with physician coleadership. Full coleadership will be impossible for most, but health systems that reach even partial coleadership will gain immense competitive and financial advantage. Like Mayo Clinic, they will rise to the top.

THE PHYSICIAN ENGAGEMENT CONTINUUM

It's helpful to start a book about physician engagement with a definition. Put simply, physician engagement exists when physicians care about the well-being of their health system and want to work with executives to solve the system's problems.

This simple definition will likely fit most executives' understanding of physician engagement, but it is too narrow for this guide. It lacks the necessary tautness of physician engagement, analogous to prongs plugged into a socket. It also misses physician accountability and decision-making authority, which are essential. We can address these shortfalls by recognizing that physician engagement exists on a continuum (exhibit 1.1):

- *Physician engagement* is the first phase—the essential first step—in a coleadership process that, if implemented intentionally and properly, progresses to physician empowerment and ultimately to physician ownership.
- *Physician empowerment* is like the unfolding of a flower. It captures the amazing transformation in confidence, motivation, engagement, and satisfaction that physicians undergo when they are given decision-making authority beyond their traditional realm of patient care.
- *Physician ownership*, the result of continual empowerment, exists when physicians begin to feel as accountable as executives for their health system's success.

Exhibit 1.1 Engagement: Starting Point Toward Ownership

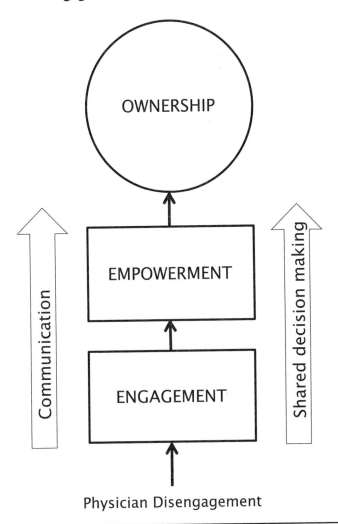

One term commonly used in health systems, but which I don't use, is *physician alignment*. It suggests that physicians are the problem, and that the solution is to bring them into line with executives' goals and views. In reality, executives' goals and views are suboptimal without physician coleadership.

A Health Leadership Lexicon

As I wrote this book, I encountered a challenge I've met while writing articles and delivering talks: namely, the lack of unambiguous words to describe ourselves as healthcare leaders and what we do.

For example, *administrator* is often used as a synonym for *CEO*. However, chief operating officers (COOs) and other executives are also frequently described as *administration* or *administrators*. Physicians in administrative roles are sometimes referred to as *physician executives*, but there is no clear distinction between which physician leaders are also executives and which are not.

For clarity, I will define three terms the way I intend for them to be understood in this book:

1. *Health system* is a hospital, or multihospital organization, and all the services it provides including outpatient services, office-based practices, and post-acute care services.
2. *Executives* are nonphysician CEOs, vice presidents, assistant vice presidents, and directors.
3. *Physician leaders* are any physicians in a formal leadership role such as the chief medical officer, medical director, department chair, division chief, and chief of service.

Physician leaders and executives become health system *coleaders* by sharing decision-making authority and goals and by treating each other as equals.

USING THIS BOOK AS YOUR GUIDE

This book is a guide to driving culture change, and culture change starts at the top. Its message is most effective when executives read the book, meet to discuss and adopt the philosophy, and then infuse that message throughout the organization. Executives at all levels should then use the book as a step-by-step guide to implementing physician engagement initiatives.

Each chapter includes a collection of pearls of practical wisdom and some tips to help executives move from understanding to action.

PHYSICIAN ENGAGEMENT PEARLS

Submerge Your Ego, Treat Physicians as Equals

When interacting with physicians, executives should avoid intimidating or appearing to be intimidated. This requires a tricky balance of humility and diplomatic assertiveness. Just as executives are used to being in charge of other executives and employees, physicians—even the most junior—are used to being in charge of care teams.

And, like executives, physicians summarily reject input they feel is wrong. When these propensities to take charge come together, there may be the potential for a clash of egos. In such situations, executives should submerge their egos because winning is really losing. The physician who loses such an arm wrestle leaves resentful, more disengaged, and less cooperative. The executive who wins validates a negative stereotype and finds physician engagement even more difficult.

Conversely, an executive who comes across as intimidated runs the risk of being considered unknowledgeable. So a balance must be struck. The best way for executives to achieve this balance is to treat physicians as equals.

Case in Point: A health system CEO faced the decision to either keep a service as provider-based (with higher reimbursement, because of facility fees) or make it office-based (with no facility fees, lower pricing, and less administrative burden).

→

The physicians in this specialty were adamant that the service should become office-based because of patient dissatisfaction with higher copays. The executives, on the other hand, preferred a hospital-based model because a conversion to office-based would entail a loss of millions of dollars for an already struggling health system. Egos clashed and the executives and physicians reached an impasse.

The CEO convened four meetings comprising the physicians and relevant health system executives. She asked the executives and physicians to not express a preformed decision. Instead, the goal of the first meeting was to collectively understand and agree to the facts; the second was to present any new information requested in the first meeting; the third was to share the different perspectives on the issue; and the fourth was to make a collaborative decision.

Barriers gradually fell as the executives and physicians learned more about the issue from each other's perspective and the physicians participated in the decision-making process.

The consensus? Make the service office-based with a commitment by the physicians to mitigate losses by increasing physician productivity and working with executives to reduce staffing expenses.

Being courteous and listening to physicians is a fundamental part of treating physicians as equals.

Case in Point: Here's an example of what not to do. A physician taped a social activism poster in the hallway outside her office. An executive had the poster taken down

→

because it did not comply with the policy for information in public areas. The physician was incensed; multiple meetings and e-mails only increased her ire. Eventually, the issue reached the CEO, who then met with the physician.

Immediately, the CEO realized that the driver of the physician's anger was a feeling of disrespect. The physician was upset that the poster was removed without discussion, that the rationale for its removal was not clearly explained, and that she was given no alternative for sharing the poster's message.

The CEO apologized and promised to handle such processes more respectfully in the future. The physician calmed down and the issue was solved to everyone's satisfaction.

As these two cases demonstrate, treating physicians as equals is more work for executives. But in the long run, not proactively doing so can generate exponentially more work—and physician disengagement.

Suppress Mistrust and Take Leaps of Faith

In many health systems with an environment of mistrust, problem-solving meetings between executives and physicians are more like poker games than team discussions. Executives privately disbelieve verbal commitments from the physicians, the physicians privately question the motives of the executives, and both parties withhold information that would weaken their positions. In addition, they bluff to advance their agendas.

To stop the gamesmanship, executives must take leaps of faith that demonstrate their willingness to trust physicians, even when experience does not support this trust. For this approach to be effective, executives must at the same time explicitly state that they will hold the physicians accountable for delivering on their promises and will rescind confidence if they fail to deliver.

Case in Point: A health system's hematologist–oncologists persistently experienced an above-average length of stay for sickle cell patients. A young hematology–oncology physician said she could reduce this length of stay if executives would only invest in more staff, space, and resources for a sickle cell day hospital—essentially an outpatient observation unit. She also committed to doing the outreach necessary to ensure an adequate volume of patients to warrant such a service.

This request came amid systemwide cost-cutting (hence the scrutiny on length of stay), and it would have been understandable for the executives to respond, "We are looking for cost savings and the doctors are using this as an excuse to use pie-in-the-sky projections to press for more expenditure." Instead, the executives took the physician at her word, while emphasizing that this leap of faith was based on their confidence in her promise.

The results were impressive. The physician reduced the length of stay by one day, grew the patient volume, and exceeded her financial projections. In the process, the physician became empowered and took ownership while the executives developed a genuine and deep trust.

Of course, leaps of faith must be based on good information. In this case, the physician was asked to develop a business plan, which was reviewed by the executives before approval. Also, executives and employees were obligated to help the physician. Even when a project is proposed by a physician, responsibility for the endeavor is always shared.

INSIDE TIPS

1. Achieving physician engagement, and ultimately ownership, requires a culture change that can only happen if the CEO and other executives want it to happen and understand their role. One approach to consensus is for everyone on the executive team to read this book at the same time and then meet to discuss a chapter at the beginning of each senior leadership meeting. Once team members agree to drive this culture change, they can influence the rest of the organization.

2. Physician engagement is hard and involves sharing some executive decision-making authority. Assess whether you possess the personality and facilitation skills to accomplish this yourself; if not, identify executives who can partner with you to help you along the way.

3. Once you commit, gear up as you would for any other culture change, such as improving patient satisfaction or employee engagement. Take stock of the existing culture through survey reports and other sources of data; set your goals for year one, two, and three, and then communicate the plan to board members, other leaders, and employees.

4. Implement easy actions for early wins to start the promotion of physician engagement and gain the attention of other executives. These may include eliminating ambiguous terms like *physician alignment*, introducing the term *coleadership*, and modifying your communications to physicians so that the words and tone demonstrate that you view them as equals.

REFERENCES

Berry, L. L., and K. D. Seltman. 2008. *Management Lessons from Mayo Clinic: Inside One of the World's Most Admired Service Organizations.* New York: McGraw-Hill.

Robeznieks, A. 2014. "Hospitals Hire More Doctors as CEOs as Focus on Quality Grows." *Modern Healthcare.* Published May 10. www.modernhealthcare.com/article/20140510/MAGAZINE/305109988.

CHAPTER 2

Bust the Myths to
Change the Culture

ACHIEVING THE ULTIMATE goal of physician ownership starts with physician engagement.

Basically, engagement is what you want from people who create or support your health system's services. Ownership is what you want from people who essentially *are* the service—that is, the physicians. Fortunately, physicians excel at ownership, as evidenced by the responsibility they take for direct patient care. The trick is getting them to also own the operational, financial, and strategic goals of the health systems in which that care occurs. When they do own those goals, as in many freestanding ambulatory surgery centers, performance improves (Ambulatory Surgery Center Association and Ambulatory Surgery Foundation 2017). When they don't . . . well, that is why you are reading this guide.

First, ask yourself whether you really want physician engagement, empowerment, and ownership. Although physician ownership brings commitment, it also requires shared decision making, and that puts many executives at varying degrees of unease. As one executive once asked me, "Why are you trying to share business decision making with the physicians? That's what administration is here for. Let physicians do what they do best: see patients!"

If that declaration sums you up, this chapter is for you because deprogramming is urgently required. If, on the other hand, you're ready to share, this chapter will help you deprogram the many executives at your health system who are not ready. Deprogramming starts with dispelling three myths that perpetuate the status quo.

MYTH 1: THE DUMB DOCTOR

The most pervasive and destructive myth is usually expressed as "doctors don't understand business," but the subtext is "doctors can't understand business." This myth underpins the usual approach of seeking physician input into already-completed business decisions rather than involving them in the formation of those decisions. Worst of all, this myth has permitted executives to undervalue and even belittle the opinions of physicians.

It's unfair to blame only executives. True, they planted the seed long ago (perhaps to ensure job security), and today many happily nurture what they sowed. But insecure physician leaders have nurtured it as well.

Case in Point: I gave a talk on the importance of physician empowerment to an association of health system leaders. To my annoyance, the only physician leader in attendance, a chief medical officer (CMO), spent the time answering e-mails or texts on his phone. From his look of disdain, I could tell he wanted me to know I was full of it.

His rudeness continued into the Q&A session, at which point (now with my blood up) I asked him if he had an opinion he wanted to share. He slowly raised his eyes and said dismissively, "Well you know, nothing you have said is realistic. We all know physicians are the problem and they are never going to get on board."

Obviously, this CMO is part of the problem.

I believe that a person who can understand the intricacies of attaching a severed limb or curing a complex disease can understand the intricacies of a hospital merger or the complexities of a balance sheet. So let's take on the next myth.

MYTH 2: THE GREEDY DOCTOR

I encountered this myth at almost every client site during my years as a performance improvement consultant to health systems. After my usual spiel to the CEO and executive team on how to empower their physicians, somebody would inevitably retort with something like, "Physicians won't do any of that unless there is something in it for them." The subtext? "Only money will motivate physicians." Every head would nod and the conversation would deteriorate into complaints about the problematic precedent of paying physicians for meeting attendance, the weakness of comanagement agreements, and the regulatory hurdles of gain-sharing—the Gordian knot formed by the undesirability of paying physicians to engage and the futility of empowerment efforts that don't include paying them to engage.

Only nonphysicians could have created this myth. Physicians know too well the free service that a healer routinely provides: after-hours phone calls and chart completions, curbside consults, rounding on evenings and weekends . . . doing what it takes to ensure good patient care. That's the sense of ownership that medical schools embed in students and residents, most of whom already have an altruistic mind-set. The weak influence of capitalism on many young doctors also explains why medical students incur monumental debt to enter pediatrics and other relatively low paid medical specialties. If physicians felt the same ownership for the operational, financial, and strategic goals of health systems that they do for patient care, the myth would die. Yet it survives because, in the absence of an approach that fosters ownership, physician engagement must be bought.

In fact, physicians aren't disengaged because they want money; they want money because they are disengaged.

MYTH 3: THE INCOMPETENT DOCTOR

Another myth underlies conversations in health systems about reducing clinical variation. The myth is couched in statements such as, "I can't believe some doctors use one suture material and others use a different suture material for the same operation." The subtext is, "Doctors don't know how to practice good medicine."

Case in Point: At the annual meeting of a health system's CEOs, one of the speakers, a corporate vice president, told a story about his mother's visits to two doctors over a couple of months. He related with incredulity how one doctor had weighed his mother with her clothes on and the next doctor, at a different office, weighed his mother with her clothes off. The room buzzed as the crowd denounced such inept medical care. They added their own examples of variation in utilization of stents, implants, and so forth—all indicating ineptitude of care.

The speaker didn't give enough details for me to justify why one physician's office chose to weigh the patient with her clothes on. However, I can say that there can be reasons for doing so (in any event, the estimated weight of the clothes can be subtracted). Regardless, the scene in the meeting exemplified for me the cultural shift that has occurred from one of respect for physicians' clinical acumen to one of disdain.

To be clear, the problem isn't the drive to reduce clinical variation. Variation is real, and it can add to costs and lower quality. The problem is the insinuation that clinical variation equals physician incompetence. With few exceptions, physicians are highly skilled and render what they believe to be the best care for their patients. Unwanted variation is sometimes caused by physician customization and shortcuts, but even when comparing the top five US doctors in a single specialty, variation exists because medicine is complex, each patient is different, physicians are trained differently, and medicine is both an art and a science.

The myth of physician incompetence is growing and has permitted some executives and their consultants to encroach on direct patient care, a trend that further disempowers and annoys physicians.

Case in Point: I watched a young consultant scold seasoned surgeons with data that showed that several of them were taking too long in surgery, using too much blood, and using unnecessary devices. The surgeons were demoralized and irritated.

Afterward, the consultant admitted to me that he had no clinical background and had only recently entered the healthcare consulting field after graduating from college with a degree in healthcare administration. Three months later, he joined a tech firm.

DEPROGRAMMING TO BUST THE MYTHS

These three myths support a culture that steadily disempowers physicians and increases the rift between executives and physicians. Executives who want to instill physician ownership in their health systems must first bust the myths.

Three deprogramming steps—relate, respect, reframe—can help bust the three myths, lead to better physician–executive relations, and support a positive coleadership management model.

Step 1: Relate

If you believe the myths, deprogram yourself by watching physicians provide patient care. I knew a highly effective health system CEO in Atlanta who every week scrubbed in with surgeons and watched them perform surgeries. His goal wasn't just to understand the work of the health system, it was to understand and relate to the physicians.

If that's too much time and trouble, periodically watch physician–patient encounters in clinics or procedures in the cardiac catheter lab. Join physician rounds, noting that this differs from the common "leaders rounding on patients." This is "leaders rounding on physicians."

Trust me: It is impossible to believe that physicians are dumb, greedy, or incompetent after you have watched them work. In fact, be prepared to be awed. It's a good thing—the start of the mental ceding of power that allows executives to share decision making in a coleadership model and foster physician ownership.

Step 2: Respect

Executives, particularly CEOs, must prohibit the propagation of myths, belittlement, and negative stereotypes. Disparagement prevents physician engagement, empowerment, and ownership. As a physician health system CEO once told me, "You can't engage physicians if you don't like them."

The top sets the tone, and healthcare leaders who condone negative comments about physicians give their executives tacit permission to disempower doctors. Leaders who make it clear that physicians are equals to executives will set a solid foundation for physician ownership. I regularly remind my executive team, including the director of business development, that our physicians know much more than we do about what business expansion strategies for their specialties will work.

Step 3: Reframe

How executives characterize the role of physicians in their health system can either feed or dispel myths of physicians being of lesser standing and capability than executives. At every opportunity, executives should describe physicians with words such as *coleaders* rather than *employees* or *members of the care team.* Even the term *partners in healthcare delivery,* though better, denotes a role limited to direct patient care, whereas fully realized coleadership includes all functions of the health system that affect the patient care enterprise.

PHYSICIAN ENGAGEMENT PEARLS

Be Fair When Taking Tough Actions

Occasionally, executives must take action that will hurt an esteemed member of the medical staff. For example, it may be necessary to fire a well-loved but ineffective chief medical officer or to cancel a contract with a respected but uncooperative emergency department group. The danger is that the medical staff will rise up and thwart the action, hindering the health system's progress and damaging the executives' credibility. Executives can avoid these consequences by first understanding that physicians are not necessarily opposed to logical actions that have a negative impact on other physicians. They spend their lives taking necessary but traumatic actions such as surgery and other invasive procedures. What they are against is unfair and disrespectful treatment of colleagues.

Medical staff view themselves as a family, albeit usually a dysfunctional one. If "family" seems too strong, they at least are members of the same tribe. This kinship is inevitable when you work together on the same patients, greet in the corridors daily, and spend hours together in the middle of the night in emergency departments, call rooms, and physician lounges. The shared experience of long arduous training in medical schools, residencies, and fellowships is foundational to this bond. Just like some families, physicians may not be close on a day-to-day basis, but they pull together when one of their own is treated badly. Whereas executives may shrug when one of their colleagues is fired, physicians take it personally, and they show it.

Case in Point: A health system in the Midwest owned two hospitals in different parts of town. Each hospital had its own intensive care unit (ICU); the ICU in the smaller hospital was led by one intensivist who had created it 15 years earlier. She had difficulty recruiting and retaining other intensivists to such a small operation, so she worked most shifts, and the remaining time was covered by a part-time intensivist and the hospitalist group. The ICU in the other hospital was much larger and staffed by a large group of intensivists. The larger ICU was more efficient, better able to attract and retain young intensivists, and widely viewed by referring physicians as providing better quality.

Executives in the corporate office soon came to the conclusion that the larger ICU group should manage and staff the smaller ICU. They met with the founder of the smaller ICU to discuss their decision and lay out their plan.

The meeting went badly; the intensivist angrily disagreed with the plan and stormed out. Shortly afterward, the medical staff of the smaller hospital voiced support for her position and against that of the executives. The situation escalated to the point that even the physicians of the larger ICU group began to question whether it was a good idea to get involved.

The medical staff reaction surprised the executives because the physicians at the smaller hospital had long complained

→

---

privately about the quality of the ICU. Many admitted their patients to the larger ICU across town.

The executives paused to get to the crux of the situation. They set up meetings with the medical staff leadership and outspoken physicians of the smaller hospital. Through these meetings, the root cause of the resistance became evident. It was not that the physicians disagreed with the plan. Rather, they felt the founder of the ICU was being treated disrespectfully.

The key detail was in the smaller hospital's history, which many of the executives did not know. Fifteen years earlier, the smaller hospital had no ICU and local physicians complained that the larger hospital, which they viewed as a competitor, never returned their patients after an ICU visit. The intensivist volunteered to start an ICU service and the medical staff and hospital supported her.

For years, the ICU met the needs of local physicians and patients. The founder was competent, hardworking, and dedicated; she was respected by primary care physicians and specialists alike. In fact, the executives were astonished to find through these discussions that for the whole 15 years, the founder had been on call nearly every day and, for the first decade, took no added compensation. Finally, in the last five years, staffing problems had led to quality concerns.

With this information, the executives took a different approach to meetings with the intensivist. They started by showing respect—by apologizing for their insensitivity and the uninformed nature of their initial approach. They discussed the history of the ICU and recognized all she had done to build the service and support the hospital and community.

$\rightarrow$

They solicited her thoughts on how and why the service had changed, and laid out their reasons for seeking a solution to ensure its quality and survival. The conversation turned to preserving the intensivist's legacy, helping her to enjoy a better quality of life, and addressing the perception of quality concerns (and potential quality concerns that she identified) rather than a drive for efficiency or a criticism of the intensivist's work.

These meetings evolved into brainstorming sessions to identify the best ways to build on her legacy with a new model that would guarantee quality and financial sustainability. This included outlining her role in a consolidated model that would protect her legacy. A new compensation package would ensure parity with the larger group's members. Finally, executives arranged meetings between her and the larger intensivist group so that she could get to know them and their care philosophy.

Several sometimes-tense discussions later, the intensivist agreed that the plan made sense and that she was treated fairly. Once her colleagues knew she had been treated as they believed she deserved to be treated, they unanimously supported the plan.

Keep Quality of Care at Top of Mind

Protecting the quality of care is, of course, a threshold requirement for gaining physician support for any major change. The bar is even higher when colleagues are negatively affected. In those cases, careful executives try to guarantee an improvement of care.

If executives involved in the proposed ICU change had promised only maintenance of the existing quality of care, the change would have been doomed at the start. The medical staff would have asked, "If the quality is going to be the same, why go through all the disruption and risk?" The idea that the consolidation would improve care ultimately gave it a chance of success.

Being able to represent an improvement in quality is particularly important when the plan is to replace services that the whole medical staff depends on, such as radiology, anesthesiology, hospitalist, or emergency department (ED) groups. Physicians will often advocate keeping such groups even when it makes no business sense if they think the change will not improve patient care.

For example, firing a contracted ED group and temporarily replacing it with locums (even when locums include members of the fired group) is generally not a good idea. During the period before a permanent group is in place, the best that executives can hope for is for the quality to stay the same, and that won't satisfy the medical staff if there was any fondness for the previous group. Deterioration in quality is more likely, so executives can expect medical staff opposition.

Smart executives make sure that a concern about quality is not an issue for the medical staff, but instead is turned into a driver of their support.

Case in Point: In a California hospital recently acquired by a larger system, a long-standing and well-liked radiology group approached the new CEO and asked for a lump sum payment and a large increase in the amount to be paid to the group annually. The rationale of the radiologists, all nearing retirement, was that the previous hospital administration had undervalued their services during the preceding 20 years and they wanted to make up for lost earnings.

After a few meetings in which the CEO tried to negotiate an acceptable new agreement, the radiologists issued an

→

ultimatum: They would resign in six weeks if their demands were not met. The CEO refused to agree to what she considered extortion and instead turned to the medical staff leaders for advice.

The medical staff agreed that the radiologists' demands were unreasonable and that the CEO treated them fairly, so they sided with her. They cautioned, however, that the quality of patient care must not suffer, whatever the solution. This warning did not surprise the CEO, who understood that simply maintaining the status quo in quality would not be enough to guarantee medical staff support if she called the radiologists' bluff. So she developed a plan to ensure even better quality, should the radiologists leave.

The CEO knew the radiology group was weak in the interventional area, so she negotiated a fallback plan with an outside radiology group that was respected for cutting-edge interventional services. The short notice made this a costly option, but it guaranteed that if the radiologists quit, the quality and range of services would be even better than before.

In six weeks, the radiologists resigned as threatened, possibly as an act of brinksmanship aimed at causing a panicked medical staff to force the CEO to yield to the radiologists' demands. The CEO reassured the medical staff that patient care would be protected, and even enhanced.

The medical staff supported her position and welcomed the change because it would lead to improved quality of care and convenience for their patients.

INSIDE TIPS

1. Write down any myths you believe about physicians, then begin deprogramming yourself using the _relate, respect,_ and _reframe_ approach. Don't try to accomplish this myth busting overnight. Instead, schedule one activity a month. For example, ask a surgeon if you can observe an operation, or the lead hospitalist if you can join rounds. Once you start seeing the benefits, increase your scheduled observations of physicians to twice a month; vary the specialties and stick to the routine. You will overcome biases and physicians will appreciate your effort to understand them and their work.

2. Ask the executives who work with you and those who report to you to read this guide, then use it as a catalyst to diplomatically change the way some of them characterize physicians. For example, if an executive rolls his eyes at the mention of a physician or sends a disparaging e-mail, respond with something like, "Remember that our success as an organization relies on physician engagement; let's always be respectful." If you diligently remind other executives and serve as an example, the culture will begin to change.

3. In employee forums, medical staff meetings, physician work groups, and other meetings, use _coleadership_ to describe the role you want physicians to play in your organization. Explain that better outcomes are achieved when physicians and executives lead the organization together.

REFERENCE

Ambulatory Surgery Center Association and Ambulatory Surgery Foundation. 2017. "ASCs: A Positive Trend in Health Care." Accessed April 26. www.ascassociation.org/advancing surgicalcare/aboutascs/industryoverview/apositivetrend inhealthcare.

CHAPTER 3

Treat Physicians as Independent Employees

WITH HEALTH SYSTEMS acquiring physician practices and hiring physicians, I have heard many exasperated executives declare that "these physicians need to understand they are employees."

Technically, that is correct. Almost 40 percent of US physicians receive a paycheck from a hospital or health system (HealthLeaders Media News 2016). But in establishing physician engagement, executives must understand that a paycheck does not make physicians their typical *employees*. Employed physicians are neither rank-and-file employees, such as marketing personnel, coders, receptionists, or nurses, nor are they independent contractors, such as consultants. Physicians compose a unique hybrid category that can be termed *independent employees*. The difference comes down to control.

Not to get too official, but the US Internal Revenue Service describes the role of control in defining employees in this way:

> Under common-law rules, anyone who performs services for you is your employee if you can control what will be done and how it will be done. This is so even when you give the employee freedom of action. What matters is that you have the right to control the details of how the services are performed. (US Internal Revenue Service 2016)

Even though health systems pay salaries to employed physicians, they do not control the details of how those physicians perform their services. Physicians have always resisted the intrusion of employers between them and their patients. As Starr writes in the groundbreaking book *The Social Transformation of American Medicine* (1982, 217):

> Patients develop a personal relation with their physicians even when medical care takes place in a hospital or clinic. In this respect, hospitals and clinics are fundamentally unlike factories. The doctor's cultural authority and strategic position in the production of medical care create a distinctive base of power.

Yes, healthcare requires a team approach, but patients come to see physicians. This is not a truism that executives should broadcast, because everyone from security guard to surgeon plays an important role on the healthcare team, but executives must keep this special status in the forefront of their minds if they are to engage with physicians correctly.

Case in Point: I heard a group of executives complain that, whereas their annual raises had been delayed because of the health system's financial challenges, some physicians had received routine market adjustments. The executives misunderstood the central position of physicians. There are no jobs, no salaries, and no raises if a health system can't retain physicians.

Perhaps the most important difference between physicians and other employees is the fact that physicians are also *customers* of health systems. When we assert that the patient comes first, we must mean that the *physician patient* comes first. Let's envision the physician–patient unit as a double

→

bubble formed by the patient and the physician (exhibit 3.1). The two are inseparable and mutually supportive—the physician and patient both want the health system to provide all necessary support to ensure that the treatment is effective and part of an overall positive experience.

Smart leadership will appreciate the value of supporting both halves of the physician–patient model because this support is good for business. If support is lacking, dissatisfaction will result. Patients and their families will seek different healthcare providers.

And here is a critical point: Most dissatisfied regular employees may stay and continue to churn out what they consider to be subpar services, but physicians will instead quietly arrange for their patients to receive care elsewhere. The bond between physician and patient is stronger than the bond between physician and employer.

Exhibit 3.1 The Double Bubble Physician–Patient Unit

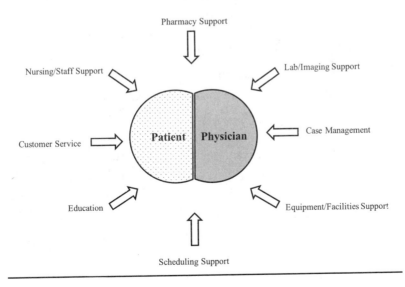

PHYSICIAN ENGAGEMENT PEARLS

Treat Physicians as Team Leaders

Executives often say that physicians are not team players, and they compare the management of them to herding cats. This characterization is inaccurate and advances unhelpful stereotypes. Anyone who has watched physicians run an emergency code, participated in a code, or even watched an episode of "ER" or "Chicago Med" knows that physicians are actually consummate team players.

What drives this mistaken belief? There is an incongruity between the role that physicians play in their world of direct patient care and the role that executives ask them to play in the executives' world of health system operations. Physicians are typically leaders. They run the code, lead the surgical team that transplants the heart, lead the team that places the chest tube, and so on. What executives see is that physicians don't do well when asked to be members of teams in which they have no leadership role or function, particularly teams led by nonphysicians.

Even when physicians serve on teams of physician peers, they can find it hard to suppress their predisposition to lead. This trait doesn't make them poor team players. After all, five health system CEOs on the same team would all try to lead in the same area at some point, and that doesn't make *them* poor team players. With CEOs or with physicians, team composition and formal leadership structure must be well planned, the goals must be clear, and there must be capable facilitation so that the role of each team member is clear.

Whenever possible, executives should give each physician member of a team responsibility for some aspect of achieving the team's goals. And when executives construct a multidisciplinary team that includes physicians, they should, in addition to giving each physician something to lead, designate the physician members collectively as leaders of the team. In other words, the physician component of the multidisciplinary team leads the others. (An example will be discussed in chapter 6, where a multidisciplinary team for an ICU cost–quality improvement campaign is led by the intensivists.)

It is important to also designate someone, usually an executive, to facilitate the team because (1) physicians are not familiar with leading non–care delivery teams and (2) a facilitator can help manage disagreements or tensions that arise in the physician cohort. If the physicians on a multidisciplinary team cannot be given individual or collective leadership functions, designate the physicians as "subject matter experts." This alternative is comfortable for physicians because it mimics the role they sometimes play as specialists on care teams led by other physicians.

As mentioned earlier, the situation is trickier when constructing a team that comprises only physicians, particularly of the same specialty and similar qualifications, such as a team of general surgeons. Here, the solution is to have the formal physician leader, such as the department chair, lead the meeting. This simulates physician meetings that would occur in a group practice.

Case in Point: Executives at an academic health system who wanted to decrease clinical variation in general surgery created a successful work group of seven general surgeons. The department chairman, a respected surgeon, led the first meeting and periodically attended follow-up meetings. When he could not attend, the chairman delegated leadership to his chief of service. The chief of service and the executives prepped the chairman before meetings and kept him updated on meetings that occurred in his absence. Although meetings were led by the chairman and his designee, a senior executive served as facilitator.

Speak Plainly and Set Expectations

Statements made by executives to physicians are often interpreted as vague, ambiguous, or even disingenuous. Aside from medical jargon, physicians tend to be blunt, even with difficult messages, whereas executives are often less direct in respect for the decision-making hierarchies of health systems; laws and regulations governing operations; the desire to protect proprietary information; and public relations concerns.

For example, a physician would be comfortable telling a patient "the biopsy shows you have liver cancer, and it has spread to your lungs," or "you have a sexually transmitted disease, and we need to have your husband tested." Executives, instead, might muddle bad news with words such as *rightsizing* instead of *layoffs*, and *streamlining* instead of *cutting services*. Even simple messages such as "I am not the final decision maker" can be hidden behind cloudy phrases such as *subject to further analysis* or *pending management review*.

Case in Point: Executives at a health system decided to implement a performance incentive plan for physicians. A certain percentage of existing salaries would be withheld and the physicians would get their money back only if they met productivity, quality, and other targets. Of course, the proposal was not popular.

In the face of physician opposition, the CEO and his chief operating officer called a meeting of the executive team. However, instead of discussing the physicians' concerns about the plan, and how to address those concerns, they simply directed executives to cease referring to the financial incentive amount as a *withhold*, because they believed the label was fueling the negative perceptions. They instructed executives to call it an *earnings opportunity*. This attempt at spin only inflamed the physicians more and the initiative flopped.

This difference in communication styles between executives and physicians leads to an erosion of trust. Executives should try to be direct when dealing with physicians.

Case in Point: A physician group placed itself and its medical office building (owned by the physicians and coinvestors) up for sale as two separate offerings. A health system's CEO wanted to purchase the group without the real estate. Her second choice was to buy both, but she was not interested in owning the real estate without the physician group. There was active competition among local health systems to acquire the group, and the CEO's lawyers cautioned her to not tell the physicians that she would only acquire the real estate if she could also acquire the group (i.e., a quid pro quo arrangement).

The physicians asked the CEO directly whether she would buy the real estate without the physicians. With her legal advice in mind, the CEO gave a convoluted answer and the physicians left the conversation confused.

The physicians accepted a different offer for their group, then turned to the CEO's health system to buy the building. The CEO told them she had no interest in the real estate on its own. The physicians said they felt deceived because their understanding from their earlier meeting was that she was interested in buying the building, with or without the physicians. So if the physicians had known she was not interested in the building on its own, she would have had a better chance of acquiring the group.

INSIDE TIPS

1. Read this chapter with other executives and discuss the role of the physician both as independent employee and as

customer. When speaking to employees, executives, and physicians, highlight the new philosophy that physicians are both coleaders and customers. Explain how the organization must put the physician–patient unit first.

2. Review your written communications to physicians to make them more plain and direct. For example, don't allow a key message—no matter how difficult—to be buried in paragraph four. Pull it out and put it as the first or second line of the memo or e-mail. Also, if you find yourself writing business jargon such as *restructuring*, *streamlining*, or *reengineering*, substitute clearer phrases such as *removing a layer of management* or *reducing costs*.

3. In verbal communications, rephrase corporate-speak, the plainer the better. This tip also applies to saying "I think," which is one way executives avoid being pinned down to a position before they are ready. Either it is, it isn't, or you can't give an answer yet because you don't have all the necessary information or authority.

REFERENCES

HealthLeaders Media News. 2016. "Number of Hospital-Employed Physicians Up 50% Since 2012." Published September 8. www.healthleadersmedia.com/physician-leaders/number-hospital-employed-physicians-50-2012.

Starr, P. 1982. *The Social Transformation of American Medicine: The Rise of a Sovereign Profession and the Making of a Vast Industry.* New York: Basic Books.

US Internal Revenue Service. 2016. "Employee (Common-Law Employee)." Updated October 4. www.irs.gov/Businesses/Small-Businesses-&-Self-Employed/Employee-(Common-Law-Employee).

CHAPTER 4

Tackle the Engagement "Whys" and "Why Nows"

WHAT IS YOUR health system's *burning platform*? You know, the particular circumstance that's forcing you to take a fateful leap. Change management experts adopted the term after a disastrous 1988 North Sea oil rig fire. When interviewed later, a survivor explained how he faced the decision of staying on the platform or jumping down into the icy water: "It was fry or jump, so I jumped" (Conner 2012).

Executives who want to jump-start physician engagement should share their health system's current burning platform as the impetus for this culture change. Communicating the burning platform will answer the "why?" and the "why now?" from disengaged physicians, and it will help them focus when they do agree to colead.

The most commonly used burning platform is financial distress because, well, financial distress is common. And where this distress exists, executives desperately need the physicians to help drive cost savings. This burning platform, presented properly, is effective because physicians are motivated to preserve the facility they rely on for delivering their patients' care.

Other burning platforms could include a credible threat of financial pressures in the future, risky projects such as implementation of multimillion-dollar electronic health record systems, or building new hospital towers.

When communicating the burning platform to physicians, executives should share all details. This is critical. When executives withhold information, they confirm physicians' suspicions that the executives want their compliance rather than coleadership and their obedience rather than ownership. Executives in financially distressed organizations often make this mistake; they avoid sharing the full depth of the financial problems or, if they do, they selectively omit important details.

Their reasons for secrecy might include the belief that physicians don't need to know certain information, the fear that full disclosure of financial weakness will cause the desertion of important medical staff members to competitors, and the concern that physicians will use the information for personal gain or leak it to competitors. I am still encountering new reasons. For example, executives of a public health system on the West Coast explained to me that the information might leak to the press and make the organization look bad to legislators and taxpayers.

The problem with secrecy is that, without full information, physicians cannot make informed decisions and therefore cannot colead. Fortunately, the fears that underpin the withholding of details are unfounded; physicians don't abandon a health system unless the quality of care has begun to suffer or it is about to go out of business. And physicians are experts at keeping confidences—it is their stock-in-trade. If physicians are told they are receiving proprietary information and are asked to keep it confidential, they will do so.

When sharing details of the burning platform, executives must define any business terms they use (such as, for example, *burning platform*). Unfortunately, it is common for executives to assume that physicians are familiar with business terms. For example, executives assume that physicians who are paid based on productivity must understand *relative value units* (RVUs). It's an incorrect assumption.

Physicians are smart, but they learned a different language than that of business. Also, they are too absorbed with treating patients to read widely on nonmedical subjects (including, sometimes, their own contracts), and they are embarrassed to ask for clarification about things they feel they are expected to know. Therefore, executives must err on the side of explaining (not in a patronizing way) even basic terms such as *full-time equivalents* (or FTEs), *indirect costs*, and *contribution margin.* Failure to do so defeats the larger message.

After sharing the burning platform, the next step is for the executives to articulate a *vision*, or call to action, that addresses the burning platform. This must inspire physicians to want to colead. From the physicians' perspective, a compelling vision is one that benefits patients. Examples of visions that are ineffective because they omit the patient benefit are "balance the budget," "reverse losses," and "ensure financial sustainability." A better vision is "to improve finances so as to allow for reinvestment in patient care." But the best visions are what I call *higher order* visions.

Case in Point: When I served as CEO of Grady Health System in Atlanta, our separately licensed children's hospital was losing $7 million per year and needed a partial building replacement that was projected to cost $30 million. After examining the options, leadership decided to merge the hospital with a private children's health system also in Atlanta. The decision was controversial because some physicians considered the private children's health system to be a competitor.

The vision (exhibit 4.1) that motivated the physicians, donors, and other stakeholders was that "every child in Atlanta who needs admission will receive the same standard of care, and that will be the standard of a [national] top-ten children's hospital." The burning platform was financial but the soaring vision was about patients.

A higher order vision is more than just a call to action; it also incorporates a strong value proposition, or benefit, for the patient. In the case of the children's hospital, the value proposition was that

Exhibit 4.1 Creating and Articulating a Compelling Vision

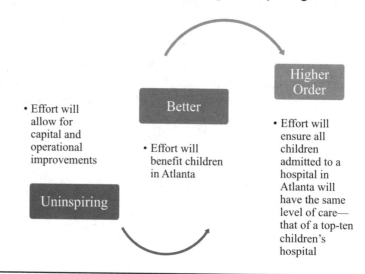

- Effort will allow for capital and operational improvements

Better

- Effort will benefit children in Atlanta

Uninspiring

Higher Order

- Effort will ensure all children admitted to a hospital in Atlanta will have the same level of care— that of a top-ten children's hospital

all admitted children would get the best level of care available. This is important. Even when a burning platform does not lend itself to a fully formed higher order vision, executives must still be able to articulate a strong patient-centered value proposition.

Case in Point: A health system on the East Coast was faced with the problem of what to do with two established pediatric community clinics that admirably served vulnerable neighborhoods but lost a great deal of money every year. Not only did the clinics consistently lose money, but they also did not fit strategically with the rest of the system, which was focused on adult acute care. In fact, the system was not even licensed to admit children.

$\longrightarrow$

Because of this lack of fit and increasing losses, the CEO and executive team decided to act. The CEO met with a local children's hospital, and a tentative plan emerged to address these issues while protecting access for the communities that the clinics served. The health system would stop providing pediatric services, but if the pediatricians agreed, the children's hospital would hire them and continue to provide the same services at the same location.

Two pediatric clinics losing money typically doesn't qualify as a burning platform for a whole health system, and this case was no different except that it was a burning platform for the pediatricians. They were proud and protective of the service they had built, so the executives needed a higher-order vision, or at least a strong value proposition, to convince the physicians of the plan's merits.

It is hard to articulate a soaring vision with a plan to exit a long-standing service, so the executives went instead with the core value proposition—the patients and pediatricians were better served by clinics owned by the local children's hospital with its focus on pediatrics, its commitment to cutting-edge community pediatric care, and the likelihood that it would not just sustain the service but would grow it over time.

It's important to underscore the fact that a value proposition must be true to be strong; physicians will see through value propositions that are wishful thinking or concocted simply to co-opt them. The executive's goal is not to create a good argument to convince physicians to support a plan. Rather, the goal is to create a solution that has a genuine short- or long-term benefit for patients and other key stakeholders.

PHYSICIAN ENGAGEMENT PEARLS

Demonstrate Your Ethics

The practice of medicine is viewed by patients and physicians alike as a noble profession. Every profession has its bad players, but the vast majority of physicians spend every day doing good and holding themselves to the highest ethical standards. Unfortunately, physicians do not necessarily view executives as being equally principled, in part because they do not view managing operations and finances as inherently noble, and because they haven't gotten to know the executives.

The executives must make it a point to demonstrate that they are equally principled and morally upright. This will increase respect and trust and help in discussions with difficult physicians. Ironically, demonstrating ethical behavior to physicians often involves dealing with the few unethical physicians in a health system.

Case in Point: A health system's top admitting surgeon was known to mistreat nurses and other staff. His behavior had worsened over time and come to include shouting and throwing objects in the operating room. Physician colleagues were intimidated, and attempts to address the behavior through peer review were ineffective. Eventually, the nurses and other staff stopped reporting the events, and the surgeon continued his abusive behavior unchecked.

A new CEO arrived and uncovered the issue while investigating low morale in the operating room. She first spoke to the surgeon and asked him to stop the behavior. When this failed, she brought the issue to the medical executive committee and reinstituted peer review. She

$\longrightarrow$

stayed involved in the process and reassured the peer review committee that the hospital would indemnify them for any rightful actions they might take. The committee recommended disciplinary action against the surgeon. He sued.

The health system's legal team not only defended the system and physicians, it also brought its own legal actions against the surgeon. When he realized the CEO and health system were serious and that he would likely lose the case, he dropped his suit and entered into a settlement that included agreeing to stop the bad behavior.

The medical staff was impressed that the new CEO had done the right thing despite the legal and financial risk of taking on this influential, high-volume surgeon. That one act established her as a person worthy of trust and respect.

As noted earlier, CEOs and executives who establish a good reputation will also find it easier to prevail in discussions with difficult physicians. This includes discussions with influential physicians who are used to getting their way and don't understand the Stark Law or antikickback statutes.

Case in Point: In the health system with the abusive surgeon, a powerful physician asked the CEO for what the physician thought was a fair and necessary increase in his medical directorship payments. The CEO refused on the grounds that such an increase would raise his compensation above fair market value and therefore would be illegal.

The physician became angry, but because of the CEO's reputation, established in the case of the abusive surgeon, he

→

accepted the refusal, trusting that she was indeed acting out of ethical principles rather than financial expedience.

Don't Insulate Yourself from Physicians

CEOs and other executives should avoid insulating themselves from physicians, including physicians who have no formal leadership roles. In health systems, executives commonly take an informal chain of command approach to interacting with physicians—that is, they interact with the most influential physicians and official physician leaders. Interactions with other physicians occur infrequently because they consider frontline doctors to be the responsibility of physician leaders and midlevel directors.

The problem with an insular approach is that, more often than not, physician leaders don't share with frontline physicians what they hear from executives or, conversely, share with executives what they hear from frontline physicians. As such, executives lead from inside a bubble, erroneously thinking they understand the wider physician body and that the medical staff understands them; in reality, they are out of touch.

I have come to consider a good day as one in which at least two of my meetings are with physicians, including those on the front lines. Getting to know most of the medical staff is a powerful tool in driving physician engagement and, ultimately, ownership.

Making a connection isn't simple. Executives will often encounter barriers to routinely meeting with rank-and-file physicians. Sometimes, resistance comes from executives' direct reports who fear that this familiarity will usurp their roles, or that their boss will hear of problems before they (the direct reports) can fix them. Some physician leaders jealously guard their exclusive access to executives. In those health systems, rank-and-file doctors worry that they will cause offense and face retaliation for meeting with executives. Even in large systems with none of these barriers, there are too many physicians for the CEO and other executives to meet with individually.

Where barriers exist, bursting through the bubble often requires a mini-change in culture. First, the CEO and other executives must establish that they intend to get to know all physicians. This is different from a passive open-door policy; it is a proactive reaching-out policy that includes meet-and-greet meetings with individual physicians for no other reason than to establish a relationship. Where the medical staff is large, executives should also attend department meetings to meet the physicians, discuss the executives' vision, and hear concerns and suggestions.

With an established routine of meeting with physicians at all levels of the health system, executives can allay the fears of their direct reports and the physician leaders by sharing, in a constructive manner, complaints they hear. If executives do this without rushing to judgment or apportioning blame, their direct reports and the physician leaders will accept the disruption to the chain of command.

INSIDE TIPS

1. Select a burning platform to communicate to the physicians and the rest of the organization. Make sure it is truly an imminent threat to organizational survival (that is, burning, not just smoldering). The general challenges of healthcare reform and value-based care aren't burning platforms, nor are narrow or time-limited issues such as a potential union strike. One way to ensure you have an issue worthy of asking physicians to rally around is to anticipate their questions. For example, for a financial burning platform, first ask yourself what the effect on finances or other metrics will be if the issue isn't addressed over the next three years. Is it an imminent threat to the whole organization? What caused the issue? Why can't it be addressed through routine management actions? Once

you have answered these questions and you still think it's a genuine burning platform, commit to sharing the details with the physicians.

2. Craft a compelling vision for addressing the burning platform. This is different than, and does not replace, the existing vision on your website. Most health systems have established vision statements that include terms such as *to become the employer of choice*. These visions were typically crafted through an inclusive strategic planning process and approved by the board. The vision to address the burning platform, on the other hand, is one that you should craft yourself and polish with input from others. To do this without seeming to break visioning convention, call it a working vision, as in one that guides day-to-day work to address the burning platform, or a draft vision, as in one that isn't official. Once you have crafted a vision, edit it to make sure it is high order and contains a strong value proposition.

3. Check your calendar for the next four weeks. Try to schedule one to two physician meetings per day, with individuals or with groups, for at least four days of the week. Begin to proactively schedule one-to-one physician meetings and attendance at department meetings.

4. Make a mental list of any potentially unethical issues occurring in the health system, such as a disruptive physician, executives engaged in nepotism, or conflicts of interest, and so on. Choose one and address it. Then move on to others. And clean up your own act if you engage in personal or professional behavior that might raise questions from staff.

REFERENCE

Conner, D. 2012. "The Real Story of the Burning Platform." *Change Thinking* (blog). Posted August 16. www.projectmanagement .com/blog-post/5755/The-Real-Story-of-the-Burning-Platform.

CHAPTER 5

Dive into the Data

THE NEXT CRITICAL step for executives trying to secure physician engagement, empowerment, and ownership is to share data about cost overruns or other problems that need to be addressed. Executives who have caught the attention of physicians with a burning platform and vision will either hook them or lose them at this stage. They must, therefore, be prepared to present the data starting with understanding the role data play in physician ownership.

I often hear executives say that "physician engagement is all about the data, because physicians are scientists." They're really suggesting that good data can be motivation enough. This is not correct. In fact, communication and shared decision making are the keys to physician engagement; data are not. The true role of data is to enable shared decision making and to help physicians and executives identify and solve problems. Failure to understand this distinction puts too much reliance on the data.

Executives who make physician ownership too dependent on data will be disappointed. Operational and financial data don't usually stand up well to physician scrutiny. Take clinical variation data as an example: Physicians are always surprised to find that the source of the data is typically not the doctors' notations in the electronic health record or paper charts, but rather transactional data from billing systems. They are dismayed to learn that the cost data are often not the actual costs from an accounting system but an approximate calculation based on cost-to-charge ratios, and that even if the data are from a good cost accounting system, it isn't practical to compare itemized costs (e.g., costs of albuterol nebulizations administered to an asthma patient versus the same costs in unaffiliated health systems across the country). Finally, physicians are irritated to learn that standard risk-adjusting of data is performed by an algorithm that assigns an illness level and complexity to their patients, rather than through a transparent and customized process determined by physicians.

Bottom line: Executives who rely too much on data also will be disappointed because creating physician ownership entails much more than just getting doctors to agree that the data accurately show a problem. Physicians can agree that problems exist without feeling any urge to help fix them.

To avoid an overreliance on the data, I begin my physician data-sharing sessions with a caveat: "The data are directional." (OK, I actually say, "The data *is* directional," but you get my meaning.) I then explain why the data are only directional. Honesty is critical.

Executives should hang a lantern on the key shortcomings of the data. But they should also mitigate physicians' concerns by explaining that peer hospitals face these same limitations. Explain that the data are directional because they do not reveal the cause of the problems; data may show that Dr. Smith used more stents than Dr. Jones but will not show why. The *why* is left to the experts, the physicians. Finally, explain the attribution problems. Whereas data often show variation in costs and quality by physician, they do not usually account for the fact that a physician may be the attending of record but may not have directed every aspect of the patient's care.

I know it is hard for executives to imagine standing in front of physicians and bashing the very data they hoped would convince them to become coleaders, but this discomfort is unwarranted. Physicians are not geeky scientists who require presentations that approximate technical dissertations. Although physicians are scientists, when listening to operational or business problems they are simply trying to understand the problem and its cause, just like anyone else. Executives think nothing of explaining to business colleagues that a piece of financial or operational data represents an estimate, a projection, or a proxy for missing information. Executives' approach to physicians should be no different.

Further, not only are estimates, projections, and proxies OK, the data don't have to be error-free. When I worked as a consultant, I was warned by more than one CEO that the data must be "bulletproof" or we (the executives and consultants) would "lose the physicians." I've found, however, that when physicians detect errors in the data, the outcome can actually be positive, as long as the executive making the presentation has correctly framed the physicians' role. The right framing tells physicians that their role is to help interpret the data, vet whether it feels correct, and suggest additional data that will help clarify, prioritize, and explain the problems that the initial data exposed. This sets the foundation for a collaborative approach to the data and any errors they may contain.

Case in Point: I recall a correctly framed data presentation where a physician pointed out a strange acronym in a list of cost categories that contributed to the cost per case for a pneumonia condition. No one, including the finance executives in the room, could explain what the acronym meant. The chief financial officer made a few guesses and suggested the group move on, but the physician wasn't satisfied.

After the meeting, the finance executives explored further and discovered that the mysterious acronym and its accompanying costs had been created by low-level finance staff to allow completion of an obsolete field in the archaic cost accounting system that, if left empty, prevented moving to the next field. The item and its costs were fictitious!

→

The doctor found an error that had been in the data for years and that even finance leadership didn't know existed. In the next meeting, the executives thanked him for improving the data by helping to identify the error.

Because the role of physicians had been framed correctly, the discovery of the error did not cause the physician to doubt the data or the empowerment process. Instead, he became the biggest physician champion for physician coleadership. Identifying the error and helping the team clean up the data was a critical milestone in his journey toward ownership.

To set the right level of expectations with physicians, it is also important for executives to understand, and to communicate upfront, that business data are not as timely or detailed as the data physicians use in their work. Physicians treating diabetic ketoacidosis will often measure blood glucose and urine output hourly, venous blood gases every two hours, and blood electrolytes every 12 hours. Executives, on the other hand, base their financial and operational decisions on aggregate data that is months old. Stating this fact proactively, before presenting the data, avoids physician disappointment.

I also strongly recommend that executives present data to physicians in a dynamic, modifiable, and "drill-downable" form, rather than in a static format such as PowerPoint. This is achieved by projecting the enterprise data warehouse on a screen and using data visualization software to make it understandable. To this end, it is a good idea to bring a data analyst to the meetings to navigate the data warehouse and answer questions. A dynamic presentation allows physicians to better analyze, understand, and accept the data.

Giving physicians the ability to mine the data in real time adds a wow factor that captures physicians' attention. This practice also provides a seldom-seen level of transparency that accelerates their buy-in.

Case in Point: Orthopedic surgeons were presented with data that showed them to have a higher length of stay than benchmark hospitals. The surgeons asked to see the specific procedures and attending surgeons, the types of patients, the treatment those patients received, the days of the week the patients were discharged, and many other views of the data. Delaying the answers until follow-up meetings would have frustrated the physicians and slowed the pace to physician engagement, empowerment, and ownership.

A dynamic setup also allows physicians to modify data in the meetings, which executives should encourage. For example, I have seen a breast surgeon request that costs of the general surgeon be displayed separately from those of the plastic surgeon, and an orthopedic surgeon ask for knee joint revision costs to be removed because it skewed his data. Allowing physicians to modify the data is a way of enabling them to make the data their own rather than "data from administration."

A well-introduced and conducted data presentation, with a data analyst present, is a big step forward in the physician ownership continuum. Physicians become excited by the unprecedented amount of detail and the ability to mine and modify the data in real time. The drill-down and modification abilities, especially, facilitate physician ownership of the data.

PHYSICIAN ENGAGEMENT PEARLS

Listen to Physicians and Give Credence to Their Expertise

Executives must listen hard to what physicians have to say when it comes to issues that affect patient care. As CEOs have told me, "Last time I checked, I don't write any prescriptions," meaning that physicians, not executives, are the experts when it comes to patients. Physicians drive the quality and costs of care. This is true, but some executives fail to apply this key understanding to their day-to-day management. For example, they ignore or override physicians' opinions when it comes to changes in patient care services. In some cases, executives don't even seek those opinions.

Case in Point: Executives at a health system in the Southeast closed a low-volume, money-losing spina bifida clinic. The decision made perfect sense from a business standpoint. The problem was that the executives failed to first discuss the plan with the neurosurgeons, one of the specialty groups that had served as consultants to the clinic patients for several years.

The surgeons knew that the patients and their families would not be able to find similar services within a reasonable distance and felt that other solutions should have been explored. They also felt it was disrespectful for the executives not to have included them in decisions regarding their patients. The executives apologized for the oversight, but the neurosurgeons remained disappointed at what they interpreted as a financially motivated disregard for patient well-being.

→

This situation damaged an already fragile relationship between the surgeons and the executives. Within six months, the executives paid out much more money than the savings gained from the spina bifida clinic closure to prevent the neurosurgery group from joining a competing health system.

Advising executives to listen to physicians might seem trite, but in difficult conversations between executives and physicians, a point is often reached where the executives stop listening. This usually occurs when the physicians become entrenched in what the executives feel is a predictable position, such as when physicians oppose closure of a service or reduction in staff. It is, however, precisely at this point that executives should lean in, raise the mental shutters, and listen harder, because when it comes to their specialties, the physicians are often right.

Case in Point: I was present in a meeting between executives of a health system and employed obstetrics and gynecology (OB/GYN) physicians to get the physicians to decrease their cesarean section (C-section) rate. Existing data on deliveries showed that the health system's rate was well above the national average, and the belief among executives was that the variance resulted from the physicians' resistance to change.

The physicians argued that their C-sections were all evidence-based, and that their patients were higher-risk because the health system was an academic medical center. The executives became frustrated and stopped listening. Instead,

→

they expressed disappointment at the OB/GYN department's lack of willingness to embrace change and contemporary practice. Not surprisingly, the meeting did not go well; no punches were thrown, but there wasn't any progress either.

A follow-up meeting was scheduled for a couple of months later. Meanwhile, the health system purchased a sophisticated enterprise data warehouse from a consulting firm. When the firm analyzed the health system's data in detail, they found that the physicians were not properly documenting severity. Taking this into account and benchmarking the health system against other academic systems, rather than against a mix of academic and non-academic systems, its C-section rate was *better* than average. The real opportunity lay in length of stay.

Fortunately, the OB/GYN physicians received the news graciously. In the next meeting, they focused collaboratively on how to improve documentation and length of stay. The executives could have arrived at this insight sooner, and with less drama, if they had listened harder, asked the right questions, and remembered that the last time anyone checked, they were not writing any prescriptions.

Develop Some Clinical Knowledge

An executive once asked me jokingly, "How come doctors can go and get MBAs and become businesspeople but executives can't just go and get an MD degree?"

This is actually a profound question. Executives should be able, perhaps be required, to get some clinical training. Executives who boast (and I have met several) "I don't know anything about hospitals, but I do know about [insert managing people, growing value, or suchlike]" can rarely be as effective in engaging physicians as executives who have taken the time to learn about the clinical work of health systems.

Case in Point: One of the most effective executives I have met could converse knowledgeably with physicians of almost any specialty. When I asked him how he came to be so clinically informed, he told me that, early in his career as a CEO, he embarrassed himself in front of surgeons at a dinner. The surgeons were advising him to buy a CT scanner that could handle extremely obese patients. One of the physicians said, "We need this particular CT scan if we are to perform fundoplications at your hospital." The executive responded, "That's all very well, but my interest lies in starting a bariatric surgery program."

His chief medical officer tried to kick him under the table, but he repeated this viewpoint several times. Eventually, a physician gently informed him that fundoplication is a form of bariatric surgery.

After this gaffe, the CEO made it his mission to buy and read as many medical textbooks as possible. Today, even seasoned physicians find his knowledge of medicine to be impressive.

Executives do not need to go to this extreme but should educate themselves clinically on their areas of responsibility rather than relying on acquiring the information passively.

INSIDE TIPS

1. Buy or create an enterprise data warehouse for cost and clinical data covering outpatient and inpatient care. Be sure the data warehouse features visualization software.

2. Designate your data analytics or decision-support group as owners of the data and the data preparation for presentations. If you don't have a data analytics group, contact similarly sized health systems for models and create one. In the meantime, the finance department can own the data.

3. Designate one or more data analysts to drive the presentations, explaining and modifying data as needed. Some consulting firms will install the data warehouse and provide data analysts for the presentations.

4. Schedule a session to introduce the data and the process to the physician leaders. Keep this presentation at a high level, keeping in mind the main goals: to show the capability of the data warehouse, explain what will be done with the data, and whet their appetites for the detailed drill-down in upcoming specialty-specific meetings (detailed in chapter 6). Although the aim is to keep the presentation at a high level, some detail is necessary. Therefore, choose one or two specialties beforehand for this. Show the data to the physician leaders for those areas before the larger group meeting. This avoids surprising and potentially offending them in front of their peers.

5. Begin to educate yourself clinically. There are many sources of easy-to-review information online and at bookstores. Some companies provide quick reviews of scholarly articles. UpToDate (www.uptodate.com), for example, synthesizes multiple articles into easy-to-understand information and recommendations. Other

useful resources are peer-reviewed articles in the *New England Journal of Medicine* (www.nejm.org) and the *Journal of the American Medical Association* (http://jamanetwork.com/journals/jama). Many physicians use these same sources to keep informed.

CHAPTER 6

Launch Cost–Quality Campaigns

ONCE ENGAGED AND empowered physicians begin to own the data, the foundation is set for them to colead efforts to address the burning platform and achieve the vision. One structured approach to developing physician coleadership, and reaping its benefits, is the *cost–quality campaign.*

These campaigns, which may be organization-wide or limited to a few specialties, focus on reducing clinical variation and operational inefficiencies. In so doing, they simultaneously improve quality and costs—what is typically referred to as *improving value.*

The working units of cost–quality campaigns are single-specialty, multidisciplinary coleadership groups comprising usually three to five physicians, one to two nurse leaders, one to two finance executives, a senior operations executive such as the CEO, a chief operating officer or vice president of operations, mid-level department directors, and a data analyst.

The senior operations executive fills three roles: first, as the final decision-maker on the health system side of the coleadership group; second, as the facilitator who guides the discussions (a professional facilitator from the outside could be seen as a referee and perpetuate an "us-versus-them" dynamic); and third, as the person who ensures the group delivers measurable results. Because the last two extremely important functions involve facilitation, I refer here to the senior operations executive simply as the facilitator. The data analyst role was described in chapter 5.

The facilitator should explain his (or her) role, emphasizing that the physicians lead the multidisciplinary group; they determine the initiatives that the group will work on and how those initiatives will be implemented.

PHYSICIANS LEADING AS COLEADERS

Note that, to this point, I have been talking about physician coleadership, and now I am talking about physicians leading. To be clear, the multidisciplinary group still makes most of its decisions jointly. However, physicians assume formal leadership of the group, with authority for initiative selection and implementation decisions, for four reasons:

1. Assigning physicians to a leadership role or function enables them to excel as team members. (I touched on this point in chapter 3.)
2. Making physicians lead and take responsibility for the work of the multidisciplinary group jump-starts their empowerment.
3. Asking physicians to lead the group demonstrates the recognition that they, not the executives, are the experts in matters of clinical variation.
4. Giving physicians this jolt of authority prevents them from drifting back into learned apathy and communicates that health system executives are serious about elevating the physicians' role.

There is little risk of coleadership becoming unbalanced in favor of the physicians because in this situation, physicians will understand and appreciate that they are leading the group alongside the executives, who will help them arrive at the best outcomes for the organization.

Because having physicians lead these groups is vital to empowerment, facilitators should not make the common mistake, born of egalitarianism or political correctness, of merely placing the physicians on an equal footing with the executives and others in the group. This leads to further physician disengagement. Rather, the facilitator must state unequivocally that the physicians lead the team. Only by making leaders of physicians will executives create effective coleaders for the organization.

The physicians also need to know that the multidisciplinary coleadership group will focus not only on care delivered by the physicians, but also on the operations supporting that care—staffing, operational routines, infrastructure, and the like. This clarification communicates trust in the physicians' ability to lead on issues beyond direct patient care, gives them an incentive (the opportunity to address operational issues that have exasperated them for a long time), and avoids the perception that a cost–quality campaign is all about criticizing and blaming the physicians.

The work of each coleadership group is to use data, combined with the frontline experience of the physicians and nurses, to identify initiatives that will simultaneously reduce costs and improve quality. The word *simultaneously* is important here because if the focus is only on cost-saving initiatives, such as reducing the number of vendors for spine implants, physicians will not be interested. If the focus is only on quality improvement, such as door-to-balloon time, physicians will be interested but the discussion may not address any financial problems.

The facilitator must guide the group toward initiatives that lie at the intersection of both quality and cost. Common examples are reducing length of stay, choosing appropriate pharmaceuticals, and reducing unwarranted clinical variation. Topics may also include changing models of care, such as the mix of mid-levels and physicians in a service, or switching between geographic- and patient-based models for hospitalists. Even investing in equipment that will ultimately reduce costs and improve quality can be addressed as a potential initiative.

Once the coleadership group chooses its initiatives, early wins are important. Early wins help physicians in the group realize that their leadership is real, and that they can truly effect change.

Case in Point: An intensive care unit (ICU) multidisciplinary coleadership group selected reduction of ICU length of stay as an initiative. The group soon realized that reducing length of stay would necessitate closing the ICU to community physicians. An open model had existed for as long as anyone could remember, so closure required changes in policies, procedures, and bylaws; meetings with surgeons, hospitalists, and other employed physicians; one-to-one phone calls with community physicians; and a great deal of fortitude on the part of the chief medical officer (CMO) and the intensivists who led the group.

The initiative worked. A widespread fear that community physicians would be offended and would stop sending referrals was not realized, and the length of stay began to decrease. The early win gave the physicians the confidence and enthusiasm to tackle other initiatives.

TAKING A PROJECT MANAGEMENT APPROACH

Facilitators should use a project management approach to measure progress toward set targets. Even a few meetings without progress can quickly cause the cost–quality campaign to fizzle.

Project management is a lot of work, and the facilitator will usually require the help of a project manager or, at least, an administrative assistant. Minutes must be taken at each meeting and a tracking tool used to ensure that initiatives, progress, next steps, responsible parties, and measurable targets are documented.

Targets must include actual dollar amounts. For example, a measurable target might be "within nine months, we will reduce ICU length of stay by one day and, in doing so, save $400,000 annually." Target numbers convey to the physicians that they are accountable (or at least co-accountable) for not just quality but also cost savings. At every meeting, progress toward these goals should be reported.

A nuance to note here is that the facilitator must keep the physicians aimed at making the changes that they directly control, such as keeping patients no longer than necessary, rather than the changes the executives control, such as reducing staffing to realize the dollar benefit from reduced occupancy. Physicians will become frustrated if they reduce the length of stay but get blamed when executives are unable to convert this to dollar savings through staffing or other adjustments.

Because the multidisciplinary group comprises only a small subset of all people who will need to be involved in any significant change, the group must invite others to the meetings as necessary and communicate effectively to the rest of the organization. For example, in the changing-the-ICU-model case cited earlier, the group invited hospitalists, surgeons, emergency department leaders, nursing leaders, and others. They also brought in the health system's communications team to ensure that changes were properly shared internally and externally

Cost–quality campaigns can quickly become very complex and logistically challenging. One campaign I helped launch at Yale New Haven Health System (YNHHS) in Connecticut comprised 24 multidisciplinary coleadership groups, many with overlapping initiatives and with monthly meetings. This is why large health systems wishing to launch systemwide cost–quality campaigns would be wise (as YNNHS was) to use formal project management experts and tools, either from inside the organization or, more typically, from an external consulting firm.

COORDINATING AND CUSTOMIZING FOR EFFICIENCY

The complexity of cost–quality campaigns also makes a coordinating structure necessary (exhibit 6.1). This structure should be customized to the health system, but the coleadership groups typically report progress and proposed changes to an executive steering committee (ESC) with the CEO, chief financial officer (CFO), chief operating officer, chief nursing officer, other top executives, and selected physician leaders such as the CMO, chief of staff, key department heads, and a few members of the medical executive committee selected by the CEO and CMO. The role of the ESC is to approve significant changes, support and guide the groups, and ensure that they are progressing toward their goals.

In large campaigns, the CMO leads a separate clinical steering committee (CSC) with physician leaders, including some of those on the ESC. When a CSC exists, the work groups report directly to it, and the CSC in turn reports to the ESC. Whether or not a CSC exists, the CMO has the final word regarding any significant clinical changes and therefore reviews all work group reports before they are reported to a higher committee.

Because some changes proposed during cost–quality campaigns will be controversial and may bring significant ramifications for the organization, the ESC typically seeks final approval for such changes from a small group of the most senior executives—the executive sponsors group, which usually comprises the CEO, CFO, and COO. These executives are kept informed about any significant work group proposals before the ESC receives the reports.

This exhibit looks like a lot of meetings, but in practice the business can be conducted quite efficiently. For example, the meeting with the executive sponsors group can be a 20- to 30-minute, high-level overview once every two weeks. The ESC meeting can simply be 20 to 30 minutes carved out of the regularly scheduled senior leadership team meetings (with additional attendees joining

Exhibit 6.1 Coordinating Structure for Cost–Quality Campaigns

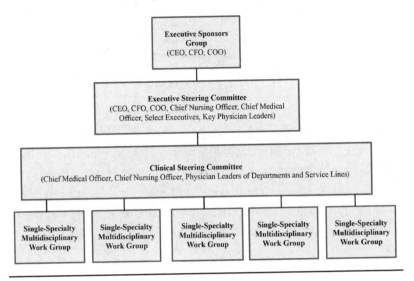

for that portion of the meeting), and the CSC can be held for an hour monthly. The benefit of this structure is that the whole effort is tightly coordinated; there is accountability and input at all levels; and the relevant stakeholders—physicians and executives—feel included in the process.

PHYSICIAN ENGAGEMENT PEARLS

Mentor Physician Leaders—Help Them Solve Dysfunction

CEOs and other executives should find subtle avenues to mentor physicians and to demonstrate the many ways executives add value to health systems. One way for executives to show value is to help physician leaders to work through dysfunctional situations that they have been unable to solve themselves.

Case in Point: An operating room (OR) executive committee, with three surgeons and an anesthesiologist, had become dysfunctional over the years because of a clash of personalities. As a result, the committee was ineffective in addressing important issues such as block time allocation.

The CEO stepped in and committed to attending the 6:45 a.m. monthly OR executive committee meetings until they were functioning effectively. She worked with the physicians to overhaul the committee, including its charter, reporting structure, level of accountability, and meeting dynamics. In six months, the committee was functioning effectively and the CEO received the following e-mail from the committee chair:

> *Thank you for your leadership and support with the OR exec committee. We have made significant strides in the right direction. We will let you know if we need your help again.*

Not only did the CEO's direct intervention help solve a critical problem for the health system, but it also allowed the CEO to directly mentor the physician leaders, modeling valuable facilitation and conflict resolution skills for them. The intervention also helped the CEO better understand the service and the surgeons.

Show You Understand the Physicians' Work

Most of the discussions executives have with physicians are clouded by the physicians' belief that executives don't understand what it takes to provide great patient care. It is therefore helpful for executives to start difficult discussions by demonstrating they appreciate the challenging and inspiring work that physicians perform every day. This approach disarms and impresses the physicians and paves the way for more collaborative problem-solving.

Case in Point: The CEO of an academic health system in Florida was faced with deciding what to do with an occupational medicine clinic that was losing money. The practice had been successful, but competition eroded its patient base and a lack of focus on operations resulted in access and efficiency problems. To make matters worse, the founding physicians were all close to retirement and younger physicians had yet to be hired to replace them.

The CEO and other executives scheduled a meeting with the physicians to discuss closing the clinic. As the meeting approached, it became clear from the physicians' frantic e-mail messages to the CEO that they believed the executives didn't comprehend the work being performed in the clinic and consequently had already made an uninformed decision to close it. When the meeting date arrived, the visibly tense physicians brought a stack of documents detailing the clinic's accomplishments. But before the lead physician could begin passing out these papers, the CEO made a few introductory comments.

The CEO, who had done extensive homework, outlined the history of the clinic and its varied functions, such as occupational medicine, employee health, and student health, and shared examples of the clinic's achievements. He described the challenges, as he understood them; he noted that although some were the results of the physicians' operational model, many were outside the physicians' control.

$\rightarrow$

He intentionally covered the work of each physician and thanked them all for their legacy and efforts over the years. By the time the CEO paused and asked the physicians if they had anything to add, they seemed relaxed; the stack of papers had been quietly pushed to one side. The rest of the conversation was collaborative and constructive.

The parties agreed to a trial period with a dramatically improved cost structure, less space, a more efficient staffing model, and a change in the physicians' model of operations.

INSIDE TIPS

1. Create a presentation to explain the "what" and "why" of a cost–quality improvement campaign. This overview may involve explaining how decreasing the cost per case while improving quality of care prepares the system for value-based care in general and risk-based contracting in particular, and also helps to improve the health system's finances. The presentation should outline core elements of the campaign: the coordinating structure, composition and function of multidisciplinary work groups, types of data those work groups will use, and project management tools and approach.

2. Present this overview to executives, and then to physician leaders. Let both groups know that an executive steering committee (ESC) will be formed to launch the campaign. If the campaign involves multiple facilities, consider engaging a consulting firm to help manage the project.

3. Create the ESC; use it to identify which specialties will launch first, and the three to five physicians per specialty whom the ESC should designate to serve on the multidisciplinary groups.

4. Convene a group session of all selected physicians and make the same presentation discussed in the first step. Be sure to communicate that participation is voluntary— tell the physicians that they have been selected to lead this important campaign for their specialties, and that you hope they will agree to do so. I have never known a physician to refuse to participate, but physicians initially might be reluctant because they are too busy. Address the time issue and reassure the physicians that meetings will be infrequent (monthly) and short (an hour), and that the effort will be staffed so they don't have to do administrative or other time-consuming work between meetings.

5. Convene the multidisciplinary groups and begin the work of the campaign. It makes sense for the facilitator to hold brief prep meetings with the data analyst and key executives before the first few meetings to ensure they go smoothly. (After a couple of months, agendas, questions, and instructions sent by e-mail typically suffice, rendering prep meetings unnecessary.) Some physicians will request their own meetings with the data analyst so they can understand the data before formal multidisciplinary group meetings. This request is helpful to the cost–quality improvement efforts, and a sign that physicians are becoming engaged.

6. If there is an area of contention that physicians cannot resolve, such as a dysfunctional medical executive committee or specialty group infighting, step in to help resolve the situation and mentor the physicians as you do so.

7. Make it a habit to place a 30-minute block on your calendar before difficult physician meetings. Use this time to educate yourself on the issue and the work of the physicians' service.

CHAPTER 7

Empower Physician Leaders

PHYSICIAN BUSINESS EMPOWERMENT is a simple but powerful concept whereby executives enable physician leaders to assume responsibility for the business management of their department or service.

At the core of physician business empowerment are monthly multidisciplinary coleadership meetings between the CEO (or senior-level designee, such as the chief operating officer), other executives, and physician leaders. In these meetings, the CEO treats the physician leaders as executives who are running their own business units. So, over time, the physician leaders take on increased decision-making authority and accountability.

Physician business empowerment is similar to a cost–quality campaign in that it promotes physician ownership through physician coleadership. Key differences are (1) business empowerment focuses on physician leaders, whereas a cost–quality campaign includes all physicians, and (2) business empowerment focuses on the business of managing and growing a department or service line, whereas a cost–quality campaign looks only at the cost and quality of clinical care.

The goal of physician business empowerment is to give physicians decision-making authority for their service lines or departments. The premise is that, with the right support (i.e., reports, data, education) and guidance of the executives, physicians can apply their subject matter expertise and frontline experience to operating and growing their domains more effectively than executives can.

This premise will disturb executives who consider the business of health systems to be their responsibility. They will be especially disturbed if they believe the myths about physicians cited in chapter 2. CEOs implementing physician business empowerment should expect resistance from executives. Some executives simply don't believe physicians are competent to run the business of health systems, and others don't believe that physicians should be given special treatment. The most common reason is that insecure executives fear a loss of power. Indeed, when implemented fully, physician business empowerment allows physician leaders to make decisions such as hiring staff, implementing new services, or changing their schedules—as long as they also meet mutually set targets and vet their decisions with their coleadership committee. So there is a shift from executives holding all the power to executives sharing power with physicians.

Fortunately, resistance dissolves when executives come to realize physician empowerment isn't a zero sum game. Executives actually become better able to effect change in the organization as physicians develop more ownership. In this way, the executives' influence or power actually increases.

FIRST, GET EXECUTIVE BUY-IN

Overcoming executive resistance is critical. If executives don't walk their CEO's physician empowerment talk, the effort will fail, and failure will worsen the preexisting physician disengagement.

Before rolling out physician business empowerment, the CEO should lessen executives' apprehension by meeting with them to share the rationale and vision for physician empowerment. This discussion should include explaining that physician empowerment will give the organization extraordinary capabilities and competitive advantage, and that sharing decision making with physicians means holding them accountable for results, which, in turn, will make the executives' ability to implement change and hit targets easier.

Also, CEOs must always invite all relevant executives to business empowerment meetings with physician leaders. For example, coleadership meetings for an orthopedic service should include the executive responsible for the outpatient orthopedic clinics, the executive responsible for the inpatient service, the executive responsible for the operating room, and a nursing executive. The CEO also should encourage executives to hold their own preparatory meetings with physician leaders before the entire group meets. This practice gives the executives ownership in the process and helps the physicians to be prepared.

Once executives understand and buy into the process, the CEO may gradually let them conduct the meetings. However, this is a large culture change effort. The CEO or designee should, at a minimum, conduct the first six months of meetings and thereafter stay closely involved to prevent the other executives from falling back into the pattern of one-sided leadership.

NEXT, CALL ON THE PHYSICIAN LEADERS

After securing executive buy-in, the CEO should introduce physician business empowerment to the physician leaders. This progression starts with choosing two or three departments with which to pilot the concept, and then setting up introductory meetings with their physician leaders. Starting small is helpful because launching monthly business empowerment meetings for all departments simultaneously is logistically difficult and labor intensive, particularly for the finance department, which generates most of the necessary reports. Also, a successful pilot helps achieve physician buy-in.

The initial departments selected for launch will vary from organization to organization, but a practical approach is to choose one or two that are financially strong and are potential engines for further growth, along with one or two that are particularly weak and need to be strengthened. Similarly, departments can be chosen based on the quality of physician leadership to include a couple with strong, enthusiastic physician leaders who can ensure early wins, and one or two with weak leaders who need immediate strengthening. After six to nine months, the physician business empowerment effort should be expanded at a comfortable pace until all departments are included.

Executives need to address four main goals in their introductory meetings with physician leaders:

1. Explain the concept and rationale behind physician business empowerment.
2. Ask the physician leaders if they want that level of responsibility and accountability. (They must be asked, and they always say yes.)
3. Identify and provide necessary support to ensure success.
4. Map out the next steps.

Case in Point: In one introductory physician business empowerment meeting I held with an employed psychiatry chair and his chief of service, along with relevant executives, the two physician leaders welcomed the opportunity to take more responsibility.

They requested several customized financial reports to better understand their department and some basic financial education to interpret these reports. The finance department set up tutorials covering topics such as the meaning of indirect costs, the meaning of contribution margin, understanding financial statements, and understanding their budget.

In addition, finance worked with the physicians to develop customized reports and also agreed to provide, under strict confidentiality, the managed care rates being paid for

→

psychiatry services. (This information sharing is necessary if physicians are to successfully colead with executives.)

Eventually, the executives supported the hiring of a business manager to assist the physician leaders as they assumed more ownership of their department.

GOING FORWARD TOGETHER

After the introductory meeting, coleadership meetings should occur monthly. As mentioned earlier, it is important that the right persons attend these meetings. From the health system side, this meeting should include the highest decision-maker possible, preferably the CEO or chief operating officer. Other executives should include the chief financial officer or designee, and the key executives relevant to the department or service.

On the physicians' side, the roster should include the physician leader, his or her second in command (such as chief of service), and possibly other physicians who take an active part in the leadership of the department. The nurse manager and a business manager for the department or service line should be included, too.

After the introductory coleadership meeting, any new attendees are introduced to the physician business empowerment concept, but the main goal is to agree on implementation goals or targets. Targets will differ by specialty, but examples include a growth target to increase the patient volume by 5 percent, or a quality target to review psychotic patients' medications once a month.

The CEO should be ready for the argument, typically made by other executives, that the departments already have goals. This is true, but most of these goals are imposed on the departments by others such as health system executives, the Centers for Medicare & Medicaid Services, and The Joint Commission; they are not set by the physician leaders themselves. Also, traditionally, only a few goals are considered to be the responsibility of the physicians. These are typically limited to quality, physician productivity, and sometimes physician-related customer service.

In the physician business empowerment model, physician leaders propose their own goals or targets for a broader set of categories, or pillars, namely quality, customer service, employee satisfaction, finance, and growth. The typical initial response from the physician leaders (apart from a deer-in-the-headlights stare) is to regurgitate current goals, such as achieving core measures. When the executive answer to this response is "but is that what you think you should be measuring?" the comeback will always be no, which should lead the physician leaders to propose new goals that they feel are important. Through this iterative process, and with guidance from the executives, the coleadership group will agree on goals and measures.

To be clear, the departments don't abandon the existing goals and measures necessary for regulatory or other legitimate purposes. Some of these goals may even be adopted into the physician business empowerment process. Rather, the concept is to hold physician leaders accountable for targets that *they* view as meaningful.

Case in Point: At a coleadership meeting, the dermatology chair and his chief of service proposed a long-standing externally set quality goal as a quality target for the year. After being challenged at that meeting to come up with a goal of their own, they returned with "decreasing the number of missing charts to less than one per session." This very busy department still used paper charts, and for years physicians had resigned themselves to frequently not having charts available from the medical records department when the patients arrived. For these physician leaders, this measure

→

was the most important and meaningful to the quality of their work.

A psychiatry group chose a more clinically focused measure: "Achieving a depression scale score of less than 10 percent, for greater than 90 percent of patients, post-electroconvulsive therapy."

Dermatology's missing chart measure illustrates that many of the new physician business empowerment metrics will require physician leaders to work with nonclinical departments to achieve their targets, while the clinical measure for psychiatry illustrates how specific and meaningful quality measures become when crafted by physicians themselves to meet the needs of their departments and patients.

ONWARD TO IMPLEMENTATION

Once members of the coleadership group have agreed on goals or targets, the physician leaders are asked to work with the executives, business managers, and finance personnel to develop plans to achieve them. For example, the psychiatry physician leaders cited in the Case in Point proposed to more rigorously implement existing physician productivity standards and to reach out to a nearby Veterans Affairs hospital for referrals. They also developed a business plan to open a private pay clinic in an affluent suburb to offset the losses from Medicaid patients on the main health system campus.

Physician leaders often need help determining targets, and they always need help implementing initiatives to achieve those targets. For example, in the area of employee satisfaction, they may need an employee engagement survey tool to determine a percentile improvement target. In implementing initiatives to achieve the target, physician leaders may need advice on best-practice routines, such as holding periodic all-staff department meetings. For financial goals, the finance department will have to help physician leaders set budget targets. For growth, the business development function will need to help them with business plans. Executives must help physician leaders to take responsibility and to succeed.

The key to the success of physician business empowerment is for the multidisciplinary coleadership group to err on the side of supporting the physicians' decisions as long as the physicians are on track to meet their goals. The CEO or designee must make it clear to the physicians that with their newfound decision making comes accountability—failure to use the privilege responsibly or to deliver on mutually set targets could end the coleadership effort for their department.

PHYSICIAN ENGAGEMENT PEARLS

Give Physicians Positive Reinforcement

Physicians are not used to receiving positive feedback about their performance. When they treat a patient, they are working to their own standards, and their gratification comes from making the right diagnoses, performing the necessary procedures or treatments, and achieving the desired clinical outcomes.

Unlike executives, physicians typically receive no structured performance evaluation based on goals, no pat on the back from bosses. Good physicians do gain the respect of their colleagues and, as a result, a strong flow of referrals. But direct positive feedback about their competency is usually limited to sporadic letters from grateful patients.

Physicians need positive feedback when they are doing good work in an unfamiliar area, such as working with executives to improve the finances and operations of health systems. In such realms, physicians can't accurately judge their own performance; they need confirmation from executives that they are doing well. Compounding this problem is that executives often assume from the typically confident demeanor of physicians that positive feedback isn't necessary. It is.

In fact, given the usual absence of financial incentives, positive feedback is one of the only tools executives have to motivate physicians to stay engaged in coleading financial and operational improvement. Without positive feedback, physicians can become disillusioned or distracted, particularly when the effort becomes difficult or time consuming.

Case in Point: At a cardiology physician business empowerment session, the last for the financial year, the physician leader started by reviewing his department's accomplishments against the targets. They had performed well, exceeding the financial, quality, and customer service goals, but the cardiologist looked tired and read matter-of-factly through the details of these accomplishments. As he did so, the executives around the table nodded occasionally, made brief comments such as "great" and "that's good," and asked a few questions. Then, just as matter-of-factly, they suggested he move on to discuss the next year's goals.

The CEO, sensing the need to give positive feedback, called for a pause and spent the next five minutes praising the physician leader for his leadership skills over the year. The CEO cited specific examples, including how the physician leader had implemented a risky growth plan, convinced colleagues to reduce costs of care, and made some tough personnel decisions—all of which led to the excellent results.

During the CEO's comments, the physician leader brightened, sat up proudly, gave credit to his team, and committed to doing even better the next year. The CEO's positive feedback was well deserved, and it was just what the physician leader needed to recommit to the effort.

Don't Just Tell, Show

Physicians prefer to see evidence before they believe—an X-ray before they believe a bone is fractured or pale mucous membranes and a low red blood cell count before they diagnose anemia. This scientific approach, combined with physicians' general lack of familiarity with the business side of health systems, means that executives who deliver a difficult message to physicians must do so with evidence. For example, when executives are delivering the message that a physicians' service needs to be cut back or closed because it is losing money, they must show the details of the loss. Although it is sometimes enough to show a high-level profit and loss statement, prudent executives will reveal much greater detail, such as what goes into the indirect expenses, how much is gained or lost on key procedures, and even how much is reimbursed by payers.

Showing physicians the details behind a controversial plan can make executives uncomfortable because the information frequently is incomplete, debatable, or inflammatory. And there is always an element of subjectivity that can be questioned by skeptical doctors. Nevertheless, this is the best approach at least until enough trust is built that the physicians will take the executives at their word.

Fortunately, the exercise of preparing to reveal details to physicians can improve the quality of the executives' ultimate decision or plan.

Case in Point: In the case of the occupational medicine clinic discussed in chapter 6, an analysis of the losses revealed that the allocation of indirect costs for space was the biggest driver, with the second biggest driver being inefficient staffing costs. Before meeting with the physicians, the executives prepared by modeling the reduction in losses that would

→

occur if the clinic were moved to a smaller space where staffing could be shared with a primary care service. They also investigated physicians' claims that the service was on a growth trajectory that might solve its current predicament.

On this point, the executives found that, although the clinic had recently signed 15 contracts with employers (to perform work physicals and other services), deeper analysis showed that the 15 contracts amounted to only 152 new patients. This level of growth provided insufficient revenues to alter the poor financial picture. However, reducing the square footage and consolidating staffing significantly improved the finances. This option ended up being chosen instead of closure. Revealing details to skeptical physicians prevented lazy decision making on the part of executives.

INSIDE TIPS

1. Ask your senior team to read this chapter. Discuss the transformative power of physician business empowerment with them to gain executive buy in. Explain their roles in the process.

2. Select the specialties to pilot for physician business empowerment, and the physician leaders and relevant executives who will attend the multispecialty coleadership meetings. The choice of physicians and specialties should be made collaboratively by executives and the CMO.

3. Meet with the physician leaders of each chosen specialty to explain physician business empowerment responsibilities and what they should expect in the first coleadership meeting.

4. Schedule the first-phase introductory coleadership meeting. Proactively communicate the goals of this

meeting, as outlined earlier, to avoid confusion or undue anxiety.

5. Make a mental list of the physicians who have been working with executives to advance shared goals. Take a moment to give them positive feedback in the form of a thank-you e-mail, written note, phone call, or meeting. Make it a habit to give physicians positive feedback when they show signs of engaging with executives.

CHAPTER 8

Communicate with Substance and Style

TO CREATE A culture of physician ownership, the CEO and other executives first must engage in true communication—bidirectional—with physicians. Frequent, strong communication fosters physician empowerment by

- dispelling executives' myths about physicians and physicians' myths about executives,
- giving physicians the information they need to be coleaders,
- building the relationship between executives and physicians, and
- ensuring that physicians can understand (beforehand) the context behind executives' decisions.

Current communications with physicians are mostly arm's-length and unreliable, although executives aren't totally at fault. Most physicians don't read broadcast e-mails or newsletters, medical executive committees don't always share what they know with rank-and-file doctors, medical staff meetings are infrequent and often poorly attended, and so on.

One reason for this problem is that physicians' day-to-day priorities differ from those of executives. For example, because of the ubiquity of hospitalist programs, the average primary care physician (PCP) thinks little about the hospital and its goals. PCPs, therefore, see little need to communicate with hospital executives. Contrast this reality with the superb communication between PCPs and the specialists involved in their patients' care.

Another reason for the poor state of communications is that physicians are busy and have inflexible schedules. Executives generally meet during the workday and can reschedule meetings, whereas physicians have patient appointments during the day that are harder to move. Even physicians' spare time is spoken for with labs to check, rounds to make, and calls to return. Executives must find varied and creative ways to reach the physicians.

Case in Point: At the health system I lead, I hold quarterly physician forums; I periodically attend physician department meetings; and I have created a physician leadership group of department chairs, with which I meet monthly in person and biweekly by phone. I hold a biannual strategic discussion with chairs and chiefs of service, and I facilitate monthly cost–quality campaign work group meetings with four key specialties and physician business empowerment work group meetings with eight specialties. I also host biweekly breakfasts with small groups of frontline physicians. These appointments are all scheduled around physicians' availability, before and after work or at lunchtime and piggy-backed onto existing physician meetings.

I even have a "Dear Dr. Andy" inbox (my daughters think I run an advice column) where anyone can write to me—anonymously if preferred—on any topic.

Despite this effort, I am not reaching even half the physicians. It's just reality: Executives must constantly seek new and better ways to communicate with physicians.

Executives reading about me facilitating work groups and hosting breakfasts might wonder:

"Does the CEO really need to be that far in the weeds?"
"Doesn't that disempower the executive team?"
"Doesn't the CEO have other, more important work to do?"

The answer to the first question is that physicians are leaders who make critical, life-and-death decisions daily. They deserve (and appreciate) being able to interact with top decision-makers. When physicians are relegated to meeting only with middle management, they become disengaged and harbor resentment at perceived disrespect.

The answer to the second question is yes, a CEO facilitator may disrupt the chain of command, but that is necessary, temporarily, to (1) change the culture, (2) ensure engagement and empowerment processes are rolled out correctly, and (3) ensure that executives do not revert to one-sided leadership. CEOs should spare executives undue anxiety by making sure the executives understand the vision and rationale for engaging physicians in this manner and including them in any physician meetings that pertain to the executives' areas.

My answer to the third question is that there is no more important work for a health system CEO than driving physician ownership. The success of everything else relies on it.

MATTERS OF SUBSTANCE

It is not enough to communicate with physicians. Transparency of information is also critical. Executives should share everything they know or, at least, avoid keeping secrets that don't need to be hidden. Without full information, doctors cannot be effective coleaders with executives. And reticence to share information often ends up worsening business problems by disengaging doctors and preventing trust.

For example, it is common for executives to withhold insurance reimbursement rates from their employed physicians because, the reasoning goes, the information is proprietary and physicians don't need to know it. Yet reimbursement rates are critical information for doctors and for anyone coleading a department or service. Executives' anxiety about confidentiality is unfounded. Physicians in private practice have reimbursement information and understand the need to keep it private.

I give employed physician leaders confidential information whenever they need it, along with warnings for discretion. I have seen this approach deepen both physicians' understanding of the business of medicine and their commitment to coleadership. True, sharing sensitive information might provoke anxiety among executives, but that's OK. If you don't feel uncomfortable about the amount of information you are sharing with doctors, you are not sharing enough.

Although transparency is critical, executives must be diplomatic in their communications before trust has been established. For example, it is a grievous mistake for an executive to criticize a physician's quality of care. Physicians take this criticism personally, which is why they avoid publicly casting aspersions on the quality of their colleagues' work.

Another mistake is to tell physicians (perhaps in the context of productivity-based compensation) that they don't work hard enough. Physicians work extremely hard and wake up every day with the intention of providing the best care. So they also take this criticism personally.

Fortunately, there are diplomatic ways of making critical points. Instead of telling physicians their quality is bad, show them how their quality metrics compare to peer organizations; then ask for their thoughts on causes and how to improve quality. Being competitive, they will work hard to address the quality issues even if they are initially defensive. And instead of saying they don't work hard enough, say that they see fewer patients per session than benchmarks; ask them to tell you the operational, patient volume, and other reasons for the shortfall.

Acknowledge that physicians are not always at fault when quality or productivity is suboptimal. In fact, poor supporting operations may make it difficult for physicians to perform at their best.

Another landmine that executives must avoid is any attempt to teach physicians about their own areas of expertise. It is impossible for a nonclinician to know more than a practicing physician about the physician's specialty. Even knowledgeable executives who venture recklessly into clinical matters can easily be viewed as arrogant.

Case in Point: A management consultant presented to a group of academic orthopedic surgeons about cost savings associated with limiting the number of device vendors. She was doing well until she remarked that "most spine surgeons can't articulate a true clinical difference between the same devices from different companies."

The spine surgeon in the room vehemently disagreed and began to list several clinical differences. It took all of my facilitation skills and profuse apologies from the consultant to prevent the presentation from completely derailing.

No doubt the consultant could have quoted a list of articles to support her assertion, but rolling about in a minefield after detonating a landmine is a total misstep. As a doctor would say, prevention is better than cure.

Another no-no is to dismiss or minimize physicians' questions and suggestions. Physicians are used to being listened to by patients, colleagues, and care teams; they can perceive dismissal of their views as humiliating or confrontational. Executives should always acknowledge physicians' opinions as valid before explaining why another view trumps theirs.

Word choice and frequent clarification also are important. For example, early in the physician ownership process, when I say the word "we" (executives and physicians), I often pause and clarify with, "I mean the collective 'we.'" When executives say "we," disengaged physicians often hear "we, the administration."

I never assume that physicians understand a business term, nor do I rely on them to ask for clarification. Executives must explain even standard terms such as *full-time equivalents*. This practice even extends to terms that one might reasonably think physicians already understand.

thought *complications* referred to physician errors rather than medical complications. So the presenter paused to restate the definitions, and the presentation went well from there.

To avoid being viewed as condescending, let physicians know at the beginning of business presentations that, although many of them may understand all the terms being used, you will err on the side of over-explaining to benefit those less well-versed in business terminology.

MATTERS OF STYLE

So far in this discussion of communication, content has been the point of focus. Style, or how one communicates, is also critical. Executives who don't recognize this point quickly alienate physicians. The most effective style for physician communication is best polished through years of trial and error, but there are ways to make the polishing process less abrasive.

First, executives presenting to physicians for the first time should always "credential" themselves. Introduce yourself, including the credentials that qualify you to speak on that topic. In the medical world, physicians defer to other physicians more (or differently) qualified than they are. For example, a cardiovascular surgeon is comfortable deferring to a neurologist for conditions related to the brain or to a nephrologist for kidney conditions.

Physicians are not, however, comfortable deferring to anyone who is less or even equally qualified. Credentialing is necessary for credibility. A chief financial officer who launches into a discussion about the overutilization of coronary artery stents will find he has launched a lead balloon, whereas doctors will listen to the same topic from an executive who has managed a cardiovascular service line.

One note of caution here: It is easy, particularly for an insecure speaker, to overdo credentialing, and physicians may misinterpret this as arrogance. Again in the physicians' world, specialists rely on less qualified physicians for referrals, and have honed the art of impressing without crushing.

When presenting to physicians, executives should also try to slip in some praise for the quality of the physicians' work. This will go a long way to disarming doctors who are cynical about executives. Doing so isn't toadyism or disingenuousness, even in health systems or specialties with low quality scores. Rather, it demonstrates respect for the challenging work physicians do regardless of scores. Such praise recognizes that the standard quality measures are imprecise, and that no matter how bad a health system is, there are individual physicians who perform miracles every day.

Praise also helps reassure physicians that the presentation is not an attack on them but rather an effort to seek their coleadership to address systemic problems. Of course, citing their awards and sharing anecdotes about them will help demonstrate to physicians that the praise is sincere.

PHYSICIAN ENGAGEMENT PEARLS

Give Physicians Incentives (Even If They Don't Ask)

In fear of gainsharing penalties and to avoid anti-kickback statute or Stark Law violations, executives shy away from paying physicians incentives related to cost reduction or revenue enhancement. As a result, executives have monetary incentives to improve finance and operations, but the physicians they rely on to colead these efforts do not.

Physicians will colead without financial incentives, although I have found that offering them legally compliant incentives sends a powerful message of teamwork and respect for their time and efforts. This is true even when the incentives are small.

I once asked a physician leader to tell me the factors he thought drove the strong coleadership in his organization. He suggested

(1) pairing physicians and administrators at every level, (2) getting both members of the dyad to agree on a budget and to speak for each other at meetings, and—most importantly—(3) ensuring that incentive compensation and goals are the same. He added that the capital allocation committee was chaired by a physician and that most of the members were physicians, a shining example of physician business empowerment.

Although this example of incentives refers to physician leaders, executives should also offer incentives to frontline physicians. I know of a physician business empowerment process that includes incentives paid to the department (not individual physicians) to fund research and capital improvements. In another health system implementing an electronic health record, physician champions received additional compensation for time spent helping the health system ensure a successful rollout. The physicians did not ask for financial incentives in either of these cases, but the executives took the initiative to construct them, in full compliance with laws and fair market value guidelines, of course.

Schedule Around Physicians' Availability

Most executives have 9-to-5 (OK, 8-to-7) jobs consisting of meetings and tasks that can often be rescheduled or cancelled if necessary. Physicians, on the other hand, typically work longer hours, with tasks and patient encounters that cannot be rescheduled.

Although most executives try to accommodate with early or late meetings, they are often less sensitive to physicians' availability than they think. One problem prevalent with executives is that unless they specifically instruct their administrative assistants to schedule around physicians' availability, the physician meetings are treated like any others. That is, they are based on the executive's availability. Also, physicians have widely varying schedules. Accommodation often requires polling for convenient dates and times, and even repeating the same meeting to ensure that every physician eventually can attend.

Failure to schedule around physicians' availability leads to a lack of attendance or cancellation of patient appointments. In either case, physicians become resentful that executives put their more flexible schedules above those of patient care.

Case in Point: A CEO scheduled a strategic planning session for 30 physician leaders to occur on a weekday afternoon from 2 to 5 p.m. The choice of the time was based on the availability of a coveted modern high-tech venue, key executives' calendars, and the CEO's mistaken belief (based on anecdotal communications) that most physician leaders had administrative time or flexibility to attend on that date. Even though the event was scheduled about six weeks in advance and frequent reminders were sent out to the physicians, only 14 of the 30 attended, and three left early to take care of patients.

Realizing his mistake, the CEO asked his administrative assistant to poll the 16 remaining physicians (and the three who left early) to find a date and time that worked for all. To facilitate their attendance, he reduced the duration of the repeat meeting to one hour and recast it as a "mini-strategic planning event." The administrative assistant was able to find a 7 to 8 p.m. time that worked for the physicians, and all 19 attended. Ironically, the second abbreviated session contributed just as much, if not more, to the strength of the strategic plan as the first session.

INSIDE TIPS

1. Assess your channels of communication to physicians, and then identify gaps. Work with the executive in charge of communications, the chief medical officer, and the medical staff office to improve the methods, and increase the frequency and quality of communication to both physician leaders and frontline physicians.

2. Take ownership for the style and content of written communications from your office to physicians. Review and edit such communications so that they are clear and strike the right tone.

3. Give feedback to your direct reports on the quality and style of their presentations to physicians, preferably right after meetings with physicians. Make notes during the meeting, then ask your reports to stay back for a five-minute debrief. Be constructive: "I noticed you didn't explain that business term and I am not sure the physicians understood," or "I would have chosen words other than 'the physicians aren't productive' to describe the problem to physicians." When your direct reports communicate well to physicians, positive feedback reinforces good communication.

4. Direct your administrative assistant to schedule physician meetings around their availability rather than yours.

5. After every meeting with physicians, check how many of the invited physicians attended. If a significant percentage did not attend, poll them to find a date and time that is convenient and hold a duplicate meeting.

6. Consider legally compliant incentives to engage physicians in coleadership efforts with executives to improve finance and operations.

CHAPTER 9

Update the
Chief Medical Officer Role

To PROMOTE A culture of physician ownership, chief medical officers (CMOs) must reject the obsolete role of "liaison between medical staff and hospital administration" and instead foster coleadership among physicians and executives so that a liaison isn't necessary. The contemporary CMO's role then becomes mentoring, supporting, and educating physicians as they take shared responsibility for the health system as a whole.

To make this transition, CMOs must first question their own beliefs, just as executives must reject deep-seated myths about physicians as dumb, greedy, or incompetent. Many CMOs successfully make the shift from traditional to contemporary, but others cling to misguided beliefs:

- *Incompatibility.* "Direct interaction between 'the suits' and the medical staff inevitably leads to friction or misunderstanding, and therefore the CMO's role is to serve as the conduit for communication." This belief perpetuates an "us versus them" culture and precludes physician ownership. Contemporary CMOs build trust between the physicians and executives; they break down barriers, squash stereotypes, and correct misunderstandings so that physicians and executives can lead health systems together.

- *Neutrality.* "CMOs should take a neutral stance when administration makes controversial decisions." This belief is founded on the misguided notion that, to keep the trust of the medical staff, CMOs must avoid being viewed as residing "in administration's camp." This neutrality actually perpetuates the notion that executives cannot be trusted and that they make wrong-minded decisions. Contemporary CMOs instead model physician coleadership by participating in and taking responsibility for health system decisions.
- *Advocacy.* "The CMO's role is to advocate for the position of the medical staff, against that of the hospital administration." This CMO partisanship often arises when the CMO reports to the board rather than to the health system CEO; otherwise the opposition is usually surreptitious. This belief also perpetuates an "us versus them" culture and fuels the stereotype of an incompetent administration. Contemporary CMOs help executives build credibility with physicians.

The harsh but true takeaway here is that, because of their unique and important role, CMOs who are not part of the solution are part of the problem. I have met many such CMOs. One on the West Coast said she refused to support the executives' desire to implement a cost–quality campaign coled by physicians. "I've already tried that and it doesn't work," she explained. "More data" was all she and the physicians needed to improve cost and quality. But after they received more data, the promised results never occurred. This CMO, like many others, preferred scurrying back and forth across the demilitarized zone rather than bringing executives and physicians together to solve problems.

HELPING TO DRIVE THE PROCESS

Contemporary CMOs can help drive the physician engagement, empowerment, and ownership process in several ways. One is to improve communication, as detailed in chapters 3 and 4. The CMO can take full advantage of all available communication channels to articulate the burning platform, vision, context for decisions, and organizational commitment to physician–executive coleadership.

The contemporary CMO also serves as the ultimate physician champion in the cost–quality campaigns and physician business empowerment process discussed in chapters 6 and 7, respectively. In cost–quality campaigns, the CMO participates on the executive steering committee, heads the clinical steering committee that coordinates all the multidisciplinary work groups, and is available to support specific work groups. In physician empowerment initiatives, the CMO is often present in a mentoring and supporting role.

The effectiveness of the CMO depends on facilitation skills, level of credibility with colleagues, and complete acceptance of the concept of physician coleadership. It's a tough job, but CMOs who rise to the occasion are the difference between success and failure.

Another key function of the contemporary CMO is to encourage, support, and mentor physicians as they assume the responsibility associated with coleadership. For example, some department chairs are not familiar with basic good management practices such as holding periodic full department meetings to listen to and share information. They meet with the physicians but not the nonphysician employees. Other physician leaders have a poor management style or are unprepared to manage their areas of responsibility. A CMO can advise and support them in their coleadership development.

True, many CMO job descriptions already include "developing physician leaders," but this point typically refers to grooming individual stars for traditional clinical leadership or executive leadership roles. Contemporary CMOs expand leadership development efforts from a focus on individual physicians to the whole medical staff.

To be successful in their role, contemporary CMOs must have progressive CEOs and executives who see the value of and do not fear true physician ownership. This is often not the case. Some consultants avoid the term *physician coleadership* because it makes the CEO and senior team uncomfortable. In those health systems, the CMOs likely feel disempowered, and physician ownership is therefore unlikely.

In short, the CMO must evolve from liaison to the medical staff, leader of quality, and driver of utilization management and length-of-stay reduction. For a contemporary CMO, the key function is to elevate the physicians to own those responsibilities and to become coleaders of the health system as a whole.

PHYSICIAN ENGAGEMENT PEARLS

Be Sensitive When Discussing Large Expenditures

Physicians rarely have budgetary authority in health systems, so they are often surprised and dismayed at the large sums of money health systems pay to maintain and improve operations. They understand expenditures for new buildings and equipment to support patient care—unless they believe simple bedside needs such as staffing are being shortchanged in favor of glitzy buildings or cool technology. When large sums are spent on initiatives they consider to be unrelated to patient care (e.g., consulting fees and renovations), they often raise their eyebrows.

Executives must be sensitive to these concerns. When dismissed or handled poorly, they can escalate into deep and widespread physician dissatisfaction. Concerns about executive spending are often not the core issue, but rather the last straw before disengagement.

Case in Point: A health system in Maryland was struggling financially. Perceived underfunding of patient care was straining executive–physician relations as well. Amid these challenges, executives decided to change the layout of the nursing stations to decrease noise and foot traffic. The physicians were not consulted, and complained that the changes made it difficult to find the nurses' charts and patients' health records. Around the same time, the hospital installed an electronic health record system. The installation was plagued with glitches, which worsened the finances and made work more difficult for the physicians.

Meanwhile, the executives renovated their administrative suites. The physicians seized on this renovation as an example of administrative excess and cluelessness regarding financial and patient care priorities. The executives countered that they were saving money by coordinating renovations. The relationship with the medical staff spiraled downward, and physicians began referring their patients to a competitor; the health system declared bankruptcy shortly thereafter.

Several problems contributed to the physician dissatisfaction. But if the executives had been more sensitive, they would have recognized the bad timing for an administrative suite renovation, regardless of any efficiencies.

A frequent challenge for executives is how to handle the issue of payments for consulting engagements. Most physicians are unfamiliar with running complex multimillion-dollar businesses and therefore find it hard to accept the need for consultants—even to help fix finances. These physicians think of how many more nurses or physicians that money could provide, or they wonder why executives are paid high salaries if they have to hire consultants to do their jobs. It is therefore critical for executives who are planning to embark on an expensive consulting project to proactively explain to the physicians why the project is necessary, why the financial outlay is reasonable, and how it ultimately supports patient care.

> **Case in Point:** During a consulting engagement kickoff meeting with physicians, a California health system CEO dropped the bombshell that one of every five dollars the health system saved would go to the consultants. Although this return on investment is standard, and not bad when the savings are real, not sharing that context or explanation with a roomful of physicians is disastrous.
>
> As soon as the CEO announced the consultants' deal, physicians began furiously texting. By the end of the meeting, the whole medical staff was aware and concerned about the executives' plan to pay the consultants a large part of any savings the physicians helped administration to achieve.

Tie Financial Decisions to Patient Care

Executives will always need to make decisions that physicians will not like. That's the nature of their job. Fortunately, those decisions can be tied back to patient care. This point is important, because enhancing or protecting patient care is what physicians care about most. Many executives forget that to credibly tie a decision back to patient care, they must first avoid taking steps that indicate otherwise.

When executives quietly tell consultants to "find us $50 million in financial improvement," physicians (who always find out about these things) perceive that the goal is to hit a financial target regardless of the effect on patient care. A better approach would be to say to the consultants, "Help us protect and enhance patient care by finding ways to improve our finances."

Also, when possible, pay a fixed fee to consultants rather than a percentage of cost savings achieved; physicians will find it hard to trust consultants to enhance or protect quality if they know the consultants are incentivized on financial metrics alone.

INSIDE TIPS

1. The CEO should encourage the CMO to read this book and participate in executive team discussions regarding its concepts. If the CMO does not buy into the need for a physician coleadership culture change, the effort will be unsuccessful.

2. Clearly define the roles and responsibilities of the CMO. This task is much easier when the CMO is new. Incumbent CMOs with well-worn behavior patterns might find change difficult to achieve. In this situation, the CEO should establish the CMO's role as part of a larger exercise aimed at clarifying the roles and responsibilities of each member of the executive team. This clarification is important because some of the CMO's roles may be better handled by other executives and vice versa. Alternatively, the CEO can simply use this book as a guide for redefining the CMO's role.

3. Work with other executives to ensure that the CMO has the training, support, budgetary authority, and shared incentives to act as a coleader with others on the executive team. This practice models coleadership for the rest of the physicians.

4. Replace a CMO who cannot or will not become contemporary.

CHAPTER 10

Learn How Physicians Think

No SINGLE MIND-SET describes all physicians. I take care with stereotypes because, as described in chapter 2, they have contributed to the myths that fuel today's physician disengagement. So I carefully draw from my combined experience as a physician CEO to characterize people who choose medicine, survive the training, and then finally get to practice. I've known many to share certain traits, habits, and mind-sets. Being aware of these physician characteristics can help executives engage doctors most effectively.

One common characteristic is intelligence. Almost any physician could complete a master's in business administration (MBA) degree if he or she so chooses. Speaking from experience, I can assure you that achieving an MBA does not exceed the challenges of medical school and residency. Not to minimize business training (or to suggest that having an MBA equates with being good at business), but physicians can understand business concepts as well as any executive—if such concepts are properly explained.

Although doctors are capable of learning business concepts, that does not mean they can understand them without coaching. They require concepts to be explained, but will grasp them quickly. Knowing how to coach physicians is important because they may feel embarrassed to ask questions. My guess is that this unfortunate trait stems from patients' expectations that physicians will have all the answers. Regardless of the cause, physicians are reticent to admit when they don't understand a business acronym, term, or concept. Executives must therefore proactively explain any terms that could be unfamiliar to physicians.

Another common trait among physicians is decisiveness. Rarely does a patient leave an office without a decision. There usually isn't the time, or patient inclination, to let a situation simply play out. Physicians are also used to making multiple decisions simultaneously. For example, when a patient presents with an upper respiratory infection, eczema, and a migraine headache, the physician usually makes all the diagnoses in the same visit, or at least orders necessary lab tests. And so, physicians become frustrated when executives fail to make timely moves on complaints or requests. Executives can prevent this frustration by setting clear expectations. Even if the decision is to do nothing, inform the physicians so that they don't expect action.

Physicians are also comfortable with revising decisions that don't work. They know that their initial diagnosis will often be incorrect, so they schedule follow-up visits or order tests. Executives conducting physician coleadership meetings must be equally open to changing course when approaches to improving quality, costs, and other challenges are failing. An executive who becomes defensive or entrenched in one plan of action goes against the logical approach of physicians and promotes disengagement. Setting measures of success and monitoring progress are critical; such measures enable the coleadership team to determine whether a course of action is working.

Because their decisions can have serious, even life-and-death, consequences, physicians draw from detailed, real-time diagnostic information (e.g., chest X-rays, complete blood counts, MRIs, CT scans). Naturally, they are dissatisfied with financial and operational information that is much less detailed. In the health system I lead, physicians express frustration that indirect costs are allocated not based on actual activity but on approximate cost drivers, such as square footage, of their departments.

Setting expectations is critical when presenting financial and operational information to physicians. As I mentioned in chapter

5, it's best to always qualify data as directional, and to be patient with any questions and frustrations that arise.

COMMONALITIES TO CONSIDER

Some traits are common to certain specialties, and executives embarking on a physician engagement culture change may find it useful to know them.

For example, because of the special needs of anxious children and parents, pediatricians have learned to submerge their egos. As a result, they tend to be collaborative with each other, with specialists who consult on their patients, and with executives. Pediatricians, therefore, can be good coleadership partners.

Emergency department (ED) physicians also are naturally good at coleadership. They are used to collaborative performance improvement efforts that are aimed at increasing efficiency, such as reducing ED wait times and improving patient survival via door-to-balloon times. They are also comfortable embarking on systemwide initiatives such as electronic health record implementations and even partnerships such as trauma networks with other hospitals. ED doctors can bring this same enthusiasm and willingness to collaborate to physician engagement efforts.

Hospitalists don't have the same experience in performance improvement efforts as ED physicians, but because over the years they have assumed responsibility for an increasing range of subspecialty patients, they have emerged as the most knowledgeable physicians about inpatient care dynamics. This knowledge, coupled with their interest in initiatives to improve coordination of care (and therefore make their work easier), makes them ideal for physician engagement efforts, particularly those related to cost and quality.

Orthopedics is another specialty that's often enthusiastic about coleadership. Orthopedic surgeons generally possess good minds for business. Perhaps business-minded medical students self-select into this field for reasons related to the work as well as the high, productivity-based compensation. They're also often ahead of other specialties (and some executives) in identifying efficiencies, particularly in the operating room. They are especially attuned to cost–quality improvement campaigns. One downside to their advanced interest in business matters is that they often will want to lead the efforts themselves without much executive involvement. True coleadership with orthopedic surgeons calls for a strong facilitator on the executive side, along with a well-organized process that adds value to whatever the orthopedic surgeons want to accomplish.

At the end of the day, physicians share a universal attribute, their all-consuming passion for patient care. To succeed with coleadership efforts, executives must explain to physicians how the goal at hand relates to patient care. The need to tie everything back to patient care also applies to performance improvement initiatives that physicians colead. So in cost–quality campaigns, I tell physicians to choose initiatives that reduce costs while improving or protecting quality. I explain that the cost reductions can benefit patients by ultimately making care more affordable.

PHYSICIAN ENGAGEMENT PEARLS

Harness the Innovation of Physicians

Executives don't think of physicians as being innovative when it comes to the operational improvement of health systems. This belief is understandable because physicians rarely get the opportunity to make operational improvement decisions. Without a doubt, however, physicians are innovators in direct patient care and medical research. Given encouragement and support, they can be innovative operationally, as well. This inclination is particularly true in their own specialties.

As Andrews (2016) notes:

> The great strength of practicing physicians . . . is their
> deep expertise about both medical needs and existing

technology. They instinctively think about how a device could work better, and they sometimes think up entirely novel strategies. That was the case with Thomas Fogarty, who invented the balloon catheter. Instead of opening up a patient to get at a blood clot, a difficult and risky operation, Fogarty came up with the idea of threading a tiny tube with an inflatable balloon into a person's blood vessel through a very small incision. The balloon could be inflated to widen the vessel's passageway and open up the blood flow.

This study cautioned that physicians are better innovators when they are part of a group with "interdisciplinary skills and a diversity of perspectives," that is, a coleadership group.

In fact, the ability of physicians to innovate on the operations and business side of medicine has been recognized over the years. In 1914, Henry Plummer, cofounder of Mayo Clinic, and Minneapolis architect Franklin Ellerbe invented the precursor of the EHR with a system of "overhead carriages on cables" to move paper charts at Mayo Clinic (Berry and Seltman 2008), and in 1970, two physicians in Arizona created the first freestanding ambulatory surgery center (Encyclopedia of Surgery 2017).

Case in Point: I have found that physicians, when given shared decision-making authority and free reign to brainstorm, find creative answers to problems that have stymied health systems for years. For example, one health system faced a continuing problem of readmissions from its nursing home to its main hospital. The hospitalists came up with the simple but creative idea of rounding in the nursing home. Emergency department visits dropped 30 percent, with a commensurate reduction in readmissions.

Because executives do not ask physicians to brainstorm innovative solutions to operational or financial problems, physicians need time to feel comfortable doing so. To ease the process, executives should invite them to engagement forums such as physician business empowerment meetings and strategic planning sessions. Executives should also implement some of the physicians' ideas, even small ones, to show that their creativity is valued.

Create Structure to Give Physicians Decision-Making Authority

Coleadership, essentially, is about shared decision making. Health systems that create organizational structures that demonstrate this commitment will experience physician engagement and ultimately ownership more rapidly than others. The physician–executive dyad structure, properly deployed, is one such arrangement, but there are other important structures as well.

Case in Point: A health system was about to implement a new EHR system. The information technology executives planned to simply adopt the EHR company's recommended implementation structure, which included nurse, physician, and revenue cycle advisory committees, all reporting to an executive steering committee (ESC). The new CEO, however, was committed to driving physician ownership and replaced the physician advisory committee with a physician steering committee that functioned at the same level as the ESC. The CEO also hired a chief medical information officer with responsibility to develop and maintain physician coleadership of the EHR installation.

The ultimate leadership body in a health system is, of course, the governing board. CEOs and board chairs should ensure that a good number of board members (at least 40 percent) are physicians to reflect physician coleadership at the highest levels in the organization. Where possible, the board chair or vice chair should also be a physician. This move sends a powerful message that the health system values physician leadership and considers patient care to be the priority.

INSIDE TIPS

1. Make it a habit to address physicians' complaints and requests in a timely fashion even if your response is that you are unable to solve a problem or grant a request.

2. When facing difficult problems, meet one on one with physician leaders and ask them to help you brainstorm innovative solutions. Be sure to give them notice regarding the topic so they can think through ideas beforehand.

3. In planning physician engagement efforts, use what you have learned in this chapter about the characteristics of different types of physicians to select specialties with which to start.

4. Review organizational structures in the health system to ensure that they support a culture of physician ownership rather than one-sided leadership.

5. Work with the board chair to identify physicians who could be nominated to serve on the board with the aspiration being that, eventually, about half the board members will be physicians.

REFERENCES

Andrews, E. 2016. "Why Doctors Can Be Good at Inventing But Bad for Innovation." *Stanford Graduate School of Business Insights* (blog). Posted November 16. www.gsb.stanford.edu/insights /why-doctors-can-be-good-inventing-bad-innovation.

Berry, L. L., and K. D. Seltman. 2008. *Management Lessons from Mayo Clinic: Inside One of the World's Most Admired Service Organizations.* New York: McGraw-Hill.

Encyclopedia of Surgery. 2017. "Ambulatory Surgery Centers." Accessed April 4. www.surgeryencyclopedia.com/A-Ce/Ambulatory-Surgery-Centers.html.

CHAPTER 11

Measure Progress to Ownership

IT IS A beautiful thing to see physicians become engaged and take ownership. I recall sitting in a physician business empowerment meeting, listening to the physician leaders of a psychiatry department arguing with executives for fewer nurses on one of their inpatient units. Yes, the physician leaders were arguing for *fewer nurses*.

This scenario shows what happens when physicians take ownership: They stop trying to simply protect what they have and instead argue for what they would want if they were the owners responsible for both finances and quality. Here, the psychiatrists had investigated each of their department's major cost categories. They concluded that overstaffing a low-acuity unit was contributing to their losses and making it difficult to achieve financial targets. This finding culminated in the unusual situation where psychiatrists decided the unit needed fewer nurses while the nurse executive maintained that the staffing level was appropriate.

Listening to the psychiatrists, I mentally checked a "good progress" box. Regardless of who was right, or the outcome, the physicians were thinking as owners. Achievements in physician engagement and ownership reflect a culture change and, as such, the measure of success for many achievements is subjective. The measure of many others, however, is objective.

ESTABLISHING TRUST

When physicians become engaged and empowered, trust is established.

Case in Point: A new CEO arrived at a health system in the Southeast a few years after executives tried to merge the health system with a competitor. The physicians thwarted the effort. Since that debacle, the level of trust between executives and physicians had remained extremely low. Well-wishers warned the new CEO to avoid attempts at any sort of affiliation with the competitor.

The new CEO started out by implementing strategies to improve physician engagement, empowerment, and ownership; after about a year, trust began to return to the executive–physician relationship. At this point, the CEO introduced the idea of choosing one of the nearby health systems (including the competitor) as an accountable care organization (ACO) partner. He took a transparent approach to discuss the need for this affiliation, including the pros and cons of choosing the competitor over other candidate organizations.

About 18 months after the CEO's arrival, the health system—with the support of the physicians—chose the competitor as its ACO partner. With trust, even newly established trust, previously unimaginable plans can become possible.

REDUCING COMPLAINTS, ULTIMATUMS, AND POLITICS

Executives in health systems with disengaged physicians typi-cally receive many physician complaints, often accompanied by ultimatums.

Case in Point: A CEO received an e-mail (edited here for confidentiality) from a physician who was unhappy about equipment in an operating suite:

> *Today, I performed a vascular procedure. The quality of the processor and monitor system is totally unacceptable and I will no longer perform procedures in this room. I request you allow me to use the digital rooms until the system can be updated.*

The complaint and request were legitimate, but the format (e-mail, rather than in person or by phone), the tone, and the ultimatum all indicated the high level of physician disengagement at the health system.

Along with a high number of complaints, there is also usually a great deal of political maneuvering . . . physicians complaining behind the scenes to board members or, in the case of public institu-tions, to legislators, and playing executives against each other. These destructive practices all result from physicians feeling marginalized, disengaged, and unable to get their grievances addressed.

So, one important measure of success for health systems imple-menting a physician engagement culture change is a marked reduc-tion in the amount and stridency of physician complaints. The improved communication and shared decision making that define effective physician engagement can quickly unearth physicians' concerns and provide the mechanisms, forums, and culture for these concerns to be addressed jointly by the physicians and executives. Thus, complaints are reduced.

To handle concerns and gauge the success of physician engagement efforts, executives should, at the end of every physician business empowerment session, ask "if there are any concerns that we (the collective we) are not addressing." Initially, this questioning will reveal additional concerns; after a few sessions, the concerns will peter out and the executives can mentally check off another progress box. And once physicians feel heard and have influence—that is, respected—they will no longer find end runs, threats, or other dysfunctional ways necessary to get their concerns addressed.

SATISFYING PHYSICIANS

Physicians who feel they have ownership and control are happier than those who don't feel that way.

Most executives have a story about a disgruntled physician who was opposed to some effort but whose attitude changed once he or she was given a leadership role for that effort. Similarly, in health systems that have implemented physician coleadership, the physicians start to feel better about their vocation; they exude more pride in, and optimism about, the organization. This happiness can be measured through satisfaction surveys. Problem is, these are not immediate and, through habit, responding physicians often dwell on what is not working rather than what is working. Fortunately, leaders who are communicating well with physicians will get a sense of the mood of the medical staff even in the absence of surveys.

EMPOWERING EXECUTIVES

When a health system empowers its physicians through coleadership, it also empowers its executives. In systems with disengaged physicians, executives have difficulty accomplishing controversial changes or achieving difficult financial targets that require the cooperation of physicians. The executives become disillusioned; either they stop trying or they work around the physicians, which only escalates physician disengagement.

But empowered physicians work with executives to implement change, and they take responsibility for making it happen. Executives realize that their ability to effect change greatly outweighs any concerns about sharing decision-making authority.

OBJECTIVELY GAUGING SUCCESS

The main reason for pursuing physician engagement, empowerment, and, ultimately, ownership is to improve health system performance.

Not only can the improvement resulting from physician engagement be measured objectively (as mentioned earlier), but that measurement also is integral to the physician engagement process itself. For example, in the physician business empowerment process discussed in chapter 7, physician leaders identify and adhere to goals in the areas of finance, quality, service, people, and growth; at the beginning of each monthly meeting, the entire group reviews progress against those goals.

At an end-of-year neurology physician business empowerment meeting I attended, for example, the physicians proudly presented that they had exceeded their financial targets by $800,000. This amazing achievement was a result of physician productivity increases and specific growth initiatives that the physician leaders had both recommended and taken accountability for implementing.

There are many other objective measures of the success of the physician business empowerment process. Some examples include reduction in length of stay and readmissions, improvement in employee engagement survey results, improvement in patient satisfaction scores, improvement in specialty specific quality measures, and growth in patient volume. Cost–quality campaigns also have numerous objective measures of success including a reduction of unwanted clinical variation, a decrease in costs of surgical implants, and a reduction in unnecessary, high-cost pharmaceuticals.

Of course, the overarching objective measure of success is the impact on the burning platform that served as the catalyst for the physician engagement culture change in the first place.

PHYSICIAN ENGAGEMENT PEARLS

Hold One-on-One Meetings

Physicians are comfortable in one-on-one meetings with executives because this is the format of the doctor–patient visit. In addition to being a familiar mode of interaction, physicians are used to the privacy afforded by one-on-one meetings to discuss confidential information.

One-on-one meetings with physicians work well for executives, too; the dynamic is less challenging than group meetings, where strong undercurrents such as egos, hierarchies of power, and peer pressure are at work. One-on-one meetings also allow executives to get to know the physicians personally and to make the physicians feel respected and valued as individuals.

For all these reasons, executives must hold frequent one-on-one meetings with physicians even with topics that have already been covered in group meetings. In the intimate one-on-one setting, even the most reticent physicians will speak their minds (in confidence). The invaluable information gleaned helps executives drive physician engagement and, ultimately, ownership in the health system.

Case in Point: At a health system in the Midwest, a large and vocal subset of the medical staff rushed to the defense of a colleague who was to be penalized (as the result of peer review) for disruptive behavior. The CEO sided with the peer review committee, and tensions rose.

The CEO decided to meet one-on-one with the main opponents to understand their concerns. She learned that the physicians were not opposed to penalties for their colleague per se. They agreed the physician was out of order and should be disciplined. The real issue was racial tension in the medical staff. The physician to be disciplined was African American, and the other African-American physicians felt that different standards were applied to the white medical staff, who were pushing for disciplinary action.

With this knowledge, the CEO could acknowledge racial tensions and reassure the minority physicians that the discipline was about doing what was right, not about race. She also committed to being involved in all future peer reviews to ensure objectivity. The physicians withdrew their opposition, and the appropriate action was taken. Without the confidential one-on-one meetings, the CEO would have missed the real concerns.

Be Viewed as Proactively Honest

One of the fastest ways to gain the trust of physicians is for them to view you as a person who believes in complete openness, or what might be called *proactive honesty*. Proactive honesty goes beyond the boundaries of just being honest. It means speaking the truth even when it is not expected or required, and even when it could lead to problems for the executives or the health system.

Case in Point: A CEO discovered during a casual conversation with a representative of a cafeteria services contractor that it was the firm's practice to prepare a cooked vegetarian dish using a small amount of pork broth to enhance the flavor. Further, the CEO learned that almost all of the cooked vegetarian options were prepared with pork broth, and had been for years. The firm explained that if the cooks didn't use this recipe, customers would not eat the vegetarian options, and providing them would be cost ineffective.

The CEO realized this flavor enhancement could be a problem for anyone who might, especially for religious reasons, be averse to eating meat products—pork in particular. He proposed that the health system and the food services firm disclose this practice. The firm disagreed, suggesting that the CEO was overreacting because the small amounts of pork broth were heavily diluted. Finally, the firm argued that disclosure would turn a nonissue into a potential legal liability for the health system and the firm.

Nevertheless, the CEO convened a meeting of the physicians and revealed what he had discovered. He apologized on behalf of the health system and pledged that all the vegetarian meals in the future would be free of animal products. While the physicians were not upset, they were surprised and impressed by his proactive revelation. They thanked the CEO for bringing it to their attention and for stopping the practice.

Although, as the food services firm had surmised, the practice turned out to be no big deal, the CEO's honesty cemented his reputation for integrity and values. He gained immense credibility with the medical staff, which served him well later in much more difficult discussions.

INSIDE TIPS

1. As part of physician business empowerment, create detailed dashboards to measure progress against goals. Review these with physicians at the beginning of each monthly coleadership meeting to keep the process focused, ensure accountability, and reinforce the benefits of this culture change.

2. Begin to schedule one-on-one meetings routinely with physicians. Unless there is a lengthy topic to discuss, 30-minute meetings are sufficient (and efficient for the physicians) and will allow you to schedule more of them. Although these are important opportunities to convey information to physicians, resist the temptation to do all the talking. Use most of the time to ask the physicians questions and to develop relationships.

3. Make a deliberate effort to show physicians (and employees) that you are a person of conviction, honesty, and values. Issues will arise that will give you this opportunity. Seize them.

4. Go forward and change the culture. Physician empowerment and ownership—through coleadership—can serve your organization well as you meet future challenges together. And everything starts with physician engagement.

About the Author

ANDREW C. AGWUNOBI, MD, MBA, is CEO and executive vice president for health affairs of the University of Connecticut Health System. He previously served as a leader of the Berkeley Research Group (BRG) Hospital Performance Improvement practice and continues to serve as a special adviser to BRG.

Before joining BRG, Dr. Agwunobi was CEO of Providence Healthcare, part of Providence Health & Services in Spokane, Washington. He earlier held the positions of president and CEO of Grady Health System in Atlanta, Georgia; president and CEO of Tenet South Fulton Hospital in East Point, Georgia; chief operating officer of St. Joseph Health System in California; and secretary of the Florida Agency for Health Care Administration. A pediatrician, Dr. Agwunobi received a medical degree from the Medical School of the University of Jos, Nigeria, and a master of business administration degree from the Stanford Graduate School of Business.

In 2005, he was named one of the 100 Most Influential Georgians by *Georgia Trend* magazine and in 2007 was named one of the 50 Most Powerful Physician Executives in Healthcare by *Modern Healthcare* magazine.